Arthur V. Meigs

Milk Analysis and Infant Feeding

A Practical treatise on the examination of human and cows' milk, cream,

condensed milk, etc.

Arthur V. Meigs

Milk Analysis and Infant Feeding
A Practical treatise on the examination of human and cows' milk, cream, condensed milk, etc.

ISBN/EAN: 9783337182311

Printed in Europe, USA, Canada, Australia, Japan

Cover: Foto ©Andreas Hilbeck / pixelio.de

More available books at **www.hansebooks.com**

AND

INFANT FEEDING.

A PRACTICAL TREATISE ON THE EXAMINATION
OF HUMAN AND COWS' MILK, CREAM,
CONDENSED MILK, ETC.,

AND

DIRECTIONS AS TO THE DIET OF YOUNG INFANTS.

BY

ARTHUR V. MEIGS, M.D.,

PHYSICIAN TO THE PENNSYLVANIA HOSPITAL AND TO THE CHILDREN'S
HOSPITAL; FELLOW OF THE COLLEGE OF PHYSICIANS OF
PHILADELPHIA, ETC.

PHILADELPHIA:

P. BLAKISTON, SON & CO.,

No. 1012 WALNUT STREET.

1885.

TO THE MEMORY OF

DR. JOHN FORSYTH MEIGS,

WHO HAD VAST EXPERIENCE IN THE ARTIFICIAL FEEDING OF INFANTS,

AND

WHO WAS ENDOWED WITH A RARE FACILITY FOR THEIR

SUCCESSFUL TREATMENT;

BY WHOSE ADVICE THIS WORK WAS UNDERTAKEN,

AND TO WHOSE ENCOURAGEMENT ALONE IS DUE ITS COMPLETION,

THIS BOOK IS

AFFECTIONATELY DEDICATED,

BY HIS SON,

THE AUTHOR.

iii

PREFACE.

MUCH that is contained in the following pages has already been published in the form of papers read before the Philadelphia County Medical Society and the College of Physicians of Philadelphia, and will be found in the transactions of these societies; but the subject has seemed to the author one of such great importance, and the diversity of opinions upon it expressed by different writers so great, that this little work is published with the hope that it may somewhat aid in placing the matter upon a more settled basis. If only some uniformity of opinion could be arrived at in regard to the much-vexed question of the composition of human milk, it would be a great step in advance toward the attainment of some positive conclusion in regard to the artificial feeding of infants. The author, after long and careful study of the matter, is convinced that human milk contains a very much less quantity of casein than is commonly attributed to it, and puts forth his reasons, and a detail of the methods by which the conclusions were attained, in the hope that in time they may be decided to be correct and be accepted. Even, however, if the subject-matter of the work only excites controversy, and in the course of time comes to be disproved and other positive and correct conclusions with regard to the composition of human milk can be attained, and thence some improvement in the methods of infant feeding made, the author will be satisfied that the work expended has not been in vain.

TABLE OF CONTENTS.

vii

INFANT FEEDING

AND

MILK ANALYSIS.

INTRODUCTION.

THAT it is desirable, from a utilitarian as well as from a moral point of view, that as large a number of the children born into the world as possible should live, is strongly evidenced by a contrast of the history of the Jews with that of any other people. Their fertility and increase, often under the most adverse circumstances, is one of the wonders of history; and they are the only people whose laws have always taught and enjoined that one of the first duties is the care of all children born. The Greeks and Romans, with their boasted civilization, —which it is now so much the fashion to admire— ordered by law, the destruction* of all deformed and feeble infants, and even, at times, of the healthy ones, to prevent too rapid an increase of the population ; and it was only toward the end of the third, and even in the fourth century of the Christian era, that the teachings of Christianity began to effect the revocation of the then existing barbarous cus-

---

* *Histoire des Enfants Abandonnés,* par Ernest Semichon. Paris, 1880.

2   9

toms with regard to infanticide. During all this time, and for many centuries before, the law and custom of the Jews enjoined the greatest care and tenderness for all children, even the sickly and deformed. That this custom did not entail any degeneration of the race, from feeble and deformed individuals reproducing their species, the event has proved ; for, while other nations have made laws ordering the destruction of all feeble or deformed infants, to prevent such a contingency, these peoples have died out and disappeared from the face of the earth, or have relapsed into barbarism, or again, like the Chinese, who are noted for their carelessness about the crime of infanticide, have remained for centuries, fossil-like, without either advancing or retrograding. During all this time, the Jews, who have pursued an opposite course, and have always manifested the greatest tenderness for their infants, although scattered over the face of the earth, have increased constantly in numbers and power, and have certainly undergone no degeneration in either their physical or mental attributes.

The historian Gibbon, in his memoirs of his life and writings, says, "the death of a new-born child before that of its parents may seem an unnatural, but it is strictly a probable event; since of any given number the greater part are extinguished before their ninth year, before they possess the faculties of the mind or body. Without accusing the profuse waste or imperfect workmanship of Nature, I shall only observe, that this unfavorable chance was multiplied against my infant existence. So feeble was my constitution, so precarious my life, that, in the baptism of my brothers, my father's prudence successively repeated my Christian name of Edward, that, in case of the departure of the eldest son, this patronymic appellation might be still perpetuated in the family." Then, after recounting how his life was a constant battle with disease until he was sixteen years of age, he tells that he believes he owed its preservation to the constant care and watchful solicitude of his aunt, and says, " I have never possessed or abused the insolence of health ; but since that time few persons have been more exempt from real or imaginary ills." Gibbon's five brothers and sister all died in infancy, but he, whose life at first seemed the most precarious of all, lived to write the history of the Roman Empire. Yet, if this man had been born during the days of which he wrote so well, he would have been slain in early infancy, or exposed upon a public highway, as too feeble a specimen of humanity to be allowed even a chance of life !

That many infants might be saved who now die, is shown by an examination of the mortality records of civilized nations. It is then seen that the relative number of deaths among the very young is enormously in excess of that in later life ; and this will, of course, always be so, for even in vegetable as well as in animal life the younger individuals are much more delicate, and during the early portion of their lives surrounded with many pitfalls in the shape of disease and accident. Still, when it is considered what an enormous proportion of the deaths of infants under two years of age is from nutritional disorders, it becomes evident that many of them must be avoidable.

The total number of deaths * recorded and tabulated as occurring in the United States during the census year of 1880 is 756,893 ; of these 175,266 were of children under one year of age, and 302,806 were under five years of age. Thus nearly one-half of the total number of deaths was of children under five years of age, and nearly a quarter of the total number was under one year of age. During the year 1883, more than one-quarter of the total number of deaths that took place in the city of Philadelphia was of children under one year of age (*Public Ledger*, Jan. 1, 1884).

These few figures seem to offer an abundant justification for such a book as this, for surely there is a crying need for the dissemination of knowledge which may lessen the mortality among young infants.

---

* *Medical News*, Nov. 25, 1882. Mortality Statistics of the United States.

CHAPTER I.

IT is unnecessary to elaborately discuss the usefulness of milk analysis, for it goes without saying that anything which adds to the sum of our exact knowledge must be useful, even if it does not bear any visible fruit in immediate practical gain. It is, however, by the acquisition of a more precise understanding of the composition of human milk alone, that we can hope for any improvement of our present methods of artificially feeding infants. Advancement in this matter might be possible by two methods only; first, by direct experiment upon infants, and second, by the acquisition of a precise understanding of the composition of human milk, which would enable us to compound a food more nearly resembling it than anything of which we have previously had knowledge. That our efforts in this direction have been thus far singularly unsuccessful does not admit of doubt, for it is universally conceded that the chances of life of an infant who has to be hand-fed from birth, are very much less than if he could be nursed by his mother or a wet-nurse. It is melancholy to think how many children die, year after year, simply because those who are most anxious for them to live do not know what to give them to eat; yet such is the fact. During all the

years that have passed, experiment upon experiment
has been made in all quarters of the world, and yet,
to-day, the opinions upon the subject are as numerous, and as radically at variance, as they have been
in the past. Experiment, then, it would seem, is
not to lead us to the desired goal, and our only
hope is that by carefully studying the composition
of human milk, and seeking to imitate it, can we
do anything to save the hundreds of thousands of
infants who are, year after year, sacrificed to our
want of knowledge.

Analysis is also useful in that it enables us to
detect any fraud that may be attempted by adulter-
ating cows' milk which is offered for sale.

That it is difficult to analyze milk correctly is
proved by the fact that, although many have attempted it, the greatest variety of results has been
arrived at, and the methods suggested have been as
various as the results attained. As the only kinds
of milk generally used in this country are cows'
milk and that of the woman, these alone will be
considered here. The analyses of cows' milk quoted by different authors are sufficiently nearly parallel, to render it likely that an approximately exact
knowledge of its composition has already been determined ; the analyses of human milk, however, are
so widely at variance as to leave much to be desired in that field. The conclusions of the various
investigators of this latter portion of the subject,
are so different as to render it certain that many of
them have hit wide of the mark.

Perceiving this uncertainty, the author, having made many analyses and experiments endeavoring to arrive at a definite conclusion upon the subject, ventures to lay his conclusions before the profession.

The method found most satisfactory—and it may be applied to cows' as well as human milk —is the following :—15 c.c. of milk must be obtained; of this 5 c.c. are discharged from a pipette into a small platinum dish, and at once the weight taken and noted. This dish is then placed in a water-bath, and the water kept at the boiling-point until the milk is completely dried, and ceases to lose weight. This, as Mr. Wanklyn points out, takes about three hours, when 5 c.c. of milk are used. (The most convenient water-bath is a deep skillet, and in this· is placed a disk of copper, with holes in it, of such a size as to hold the platinum dishes to be used, the whole being floated upon copper air-chambers soldered to the under side of the disk. This apparatus may be left for hours in the bath without any watching, and yet the platinum dishes are constantly immersed in the boiling water.) As soon as the weight becomes constant, it must be noted, and the contents are then incinerated, best over a blast-flame, and the weight again noted. (In incinerating, the heat used must at first be moderate, and then gradually increased.) This gives, by the difference in weight before and after drying, the water lost; by subtracting the weight of the dish from the total weight after drying, the total solids; by subtracting the weight of the dish from the total weight after incinerating, the ash is ascertained ; and, finally, by the difference in weight after drying and after incineration, the weight of solids not ash is ascertained. This last weight, however, does not enter into the final calculation, and is of no value except as a check to correct possible errors.

At the same time that the first 5 c.c. are weighed, 10 c.c. must be weighed in another dish, care being taken, of course, that the weight is exactly twice that of the 5 c.c. This is poured into a high, narrow bottle (the ordinary 100 c.c. graduated bottle answers the purpose), and 20 c.c. of distilled water added, this being used to wash all the milk from the vessel in which it was weighed into the bottle. To this are now added 20 c.c. of ether. The bottle must then be tightly stoppered and agitated violently for five minutes ; 20 c.c. of alcohol are then added, and it is agitated for five minutes more. If it is then set down for a few minutes, the contents will be found to have separated into two layers ; on top will be found ether, containing fat in solution, and below will be a mixture of part of the ether, the alcohol, and the water, containing coagulated casein in suspension and the sugar in solution. The ethereal solution, which is on top, is then drawn off with a pipette, as nearly as can be done without disturbing the lower layer ; 5 c.c. of ether are poured on to mix with what fat is left, and this drawn off. Ether should be poured on and drawn off five times, 5 c.c. being used each time, so as to remove all the fat. The ethereal solution of fat is now dried over warm water, and finally, for a few minutes, over boiling water ; the resulting weight—that of the dish being deducted— is, of course, the weight of the fat. There is now left in the bottle the sugar and casein, with the salts. The contents are carefully washed into a large platinum dish, and dried over the water-bath. The dried residue is treated with boiling water, and the dish and contents placed aside to settle. The undissolved casein soon settles to the bottom, and the clear solution of sugar is poured off. The solution of sugar is now again dried, and the same process repeated, the sediment being added to that which was obtained before. This must be done four or five times, until it is found that when boiling water is poured upon the dried sugar it dissolves completely, no flocculi of casein being seen in the solution. The casein residue is then, after being dried, treated once or twice with boiling water, to wash out any sugar that may have been left in it, care being taken that none of the solid casein is poured off with the matter dissolved. This sugar is added to that formerly obtained, and the two substances are then ready for the final drying, which must be done over the water-bath, and continued until they cease to lose weight sensibly. The two residues are then incinerated over the blast-flame, and the loss in the burning gives the weights of the casein and sugar.

In calculating results, it is easiest to bring the

amount of each constituent up to what is contained
in 100 c.c. This is done by multiplying the amounts
of water and ash by twenty, as they are arrived at
by the use of 5 c.c., and those of fat, casein, and
sugar by ten, as they are arrived at by the use of
10 c.c. of milk. The sum of the amounts of the
different constituents will be found to be, from one
hundred and one, to one hundred and three. A use
of the simple rule of three enables one easily from
this to calculate the quantities in parts of one hundred.

A comparison of the sum arrived at as above,
with the weight of the original 5 c.c. of milk, multiplied by twenty, to obtain the weight of 100 c.c. of
milk shows the error ; there being necessarily a slight
loss, or sometimes an excess, owing to imperfect drying of the sugar or casein in the second part of the
process. The error is always very slight, if proper
care has been exercised in the manipulations. Any
analysis in which it amounts to as much as one-half
of one per cent., particularly if there is excess and not
loss, should be at once thrown out, for excess can only
occur from carelessness. In an analysis carefully carried out by this process the usual error is from one-
to two-tenths of one per cent., and any error larger
than this is due to carelessness in manipulation. A
very common source of error is imperfect drying of
the sugar residue in the second part of the analysis,
and great care and patience must consequently be
exercised during this part of the process. The sugar
residue must be kept constantly in the water-bath,

and the water in a state of active ebullition until the weight becomes absolutely constant, and this usually takes from twenty to twenty-four hours. In analyzing human milk by this process, there is about seven-tenths of a gram of sugar to be dried, and, consequently, the drying takes much longer than if cows' milk is analyzed, when only about five-tenths of a gram are dealt with. For the reason that sugar is so difficult to dry perfectly, the water-bath apparatus described has been found invaluable, as by its use the dish of sugar can be kept immersed to an even depth in the boiling water as long as desired, for, as evaporation takes place and the water sinks lower and lower in the vessel, the dish, which is floated upon its surface, sinks too, whereas with the ordinary water-baths, as soon as the water evaporates a little, the platinum dish is left by the water and is merely exposed to the heat of the steam, which, in a vessel with a loose cover, does not amount to anything like 100° C. In the second portion of the analysis, after the fat has been removed by means of the ether and alcohol, care should be taken, when the remaining casein and sugar with salts, are put in the platinum dish to be dried, previous to the treatment with boiling water for their separation, that the drying is thorough. It is not necessary to continue the drying until the weight becomes absolutely constant, but the dish should be kept in the water-bath for at least three or four hours, as it will be found that the separation of the two elements is much easier, if the drying has been continued a good many hours. Long drying renders the casein almost absolutely insoluble; it becomes a hard, yellowish, horny mass, which will not dissolve even in a strong solution of caustic soda.

The effect produced in different specimens of human milk, when the ether and alcohol have been added and the liquid agitated as described, is by no means uniform. There is always, after the bottle has been set aside for a few minutes, the clear ethereal solution of fat on top, and this may be more or less yellowish in hue. It may be said here that the color of neither human nor cows' milk is a test of its richness in fat, for it is often found that a very pale milk will contain a large amount of pale fat, while, on the contrary, an unusually yellow milk may not contain more than the average amount. In the lower stratum of liquid, however, the effect is variable, sometimes quite heavy coagula, much like those produced when cows' milk is subjected to the process, are at once seen, which settle to the bottom in a thick, white, cheesy-looking mass, leaving a slightly colored fluid above, with perhaps a few minute curds sticking to the sides of the glass vessel and at the top of the lower stratum of liquid. Again, the coagulation takes place in the form of a very fine net-work, which can be distinctly seen through the sides of the glass, and which either remains suspended or sinks to the bottom only very slowly. Sometimes, when the net-work appearance is very marked and no heavy coagula at all have been produced, the solid portion remains permanently evenly distributed through the fluid, from the lower part of the ethereal solution, where the meshes can be distinctly seen, if the fluid is set in gentle motion, to the bottom of the bottle. Even after days, there may be no disposition to the formation of a sediment. The effect produced reminds one strongly of the appearance of a dishful of fine soap-bubbles, except, of course, that the meshes of the net-work in milk are infinitely smaller, and are permanent, and filled with a liquid instead of air, as in the case of the soap-bubbles. Why this difference in the coagulability exists, when milk is exposed, under the same circumstances, to the action of fixed quantities of the same reagents, cannot at present be explained. The same difference in the coagulation has been noticed in examining by the same process the artificial food presently to be described. It is not due wholly to the amount of the coagulable element (casein), for it has often been found that a specimen which showed the fine net-work coagulation contained an average quantity of the coagulable element when the analysis was, later, finished. At present, as already observed, no satisfactory explanation of this phenomenon is at hand, but it does not seem unlikely that it is due, in some way, to the degree of alkalinity of the milk examined.

The method suggested possesses many advantages ; the water and ash are determined by the old processes ; the mode of separating the fat, however, is a new one, and is susceptible of rapid application, and is more exact than the old way of extracting it with ether from the solid residue. The amount of fat in any given sample of milk can be determined in at most from half an hour to an hour. The idea of separating the fat by means of ether and alcohol was suggested by the perusal of an article by Ed. J. Hallock (*American Journal of Pharmacy*, October 1, 1874). The use of the reagents in the proportions suggested by him, however, fails to effect the purpose, as any one can see who will try the process; for the oil-globules are set free instead of being dissolved in ether, as happens when the proportions recommended are used, and they only partially rise to the top, many becoming entangled in the meshes of the coagulated casein and remaining thus distributed through the fluid. The method proposed also extracts the fat more perfectly than that used by chemists generally, of extracting it with ether from the dried residue. This has been proved by actual experiment, two samples of the same milk being taken, when the fat was extracted from the dried residue of 10 c.c. of milk, 270 milli-grammes only were obtained, whereas the ether-alcohol method gave 305 milligrammes. This difference is large enough to be a matter of great importance where such small quantities are used, as is usually the case in milk analysis.

The separation of the casein and sugar by simply dissolving the sugar in water and allowing the casein, which the drying has rendered insoluble, to go to the bottom as a sediment, and then pouring off the clear solution, may seem a return to old and crude methods. Filters, however, are very objectionable in dealing with casein ; first, because they allow considerable portions to pass through them, and, second, because the filter often becomes so clogged with the fine particles that the sugar solution can no longer pass through, or passes so slowly that the substances are lessened in quantity by decomposition before the filtration process is completed. Filters, therefore, should be discarded as unfit for use in milk analysis. This subject, however, will be more fully discussed in a future chapter.

The reason why five cubic centimetres are weighed out for the first portion of the analysis and ten for the second, instead of taking five and then ten grams, is because it affords an easy way of managing the error which must always occur to a greater or less extent in every chemical analysis. When the amount of each of the elements has been determined and the sum added up, it will usually be found that there has been a small loss (the error will sometimes be a slight amount in excess, owing to imperfect drying), and this may be disregarded, the sum being, by the simple rule of proportion, reduced to parts of one hundred. The amount of error may then be easily stated with each analysis ; and yet the analysis looks much better, and is much more easily managed, if it is thus made to appear exact. This seems, too, a perfectly fair method of statement of results, if the error is given in each case. The following explains the method of calculation. After finishing an analysis, the following weights were obtained:—

Water	. 91.54		89.0380 +		89.038
Fat . .	. 2.48 reduced by	⎫	2.4122 +	⎫	2.412
Casein	. .75 rule of pro-	⎬ =	.7294 +	⎬ =	.729
Sugar	. 7.92 portion	⎭	7.7035 +	⎭	7.704
Ash . .	.12		.1167 +		.117
	102.81				100.000

The weight of the 10 c.c. of milk used in the second portion of this analysis was 10.286 grams, which would make the weight of 100 c.c. = 102.86 grams; the loss, therefore, was .05 gram. This multiplied by 100 and divided by 102.86, the original weight, to get the percentage, gives .048, which shows the error in the analysis to be a loss of forty-eight thousandths of one per cent.

In cream analysis the method is invaluable, as it offers a means of checking, partially at any rate, any error, which may arise from imperfection in the drying, which is the difficult part in analyses carried out by the old method; of extracting the fat with ether from the dried residue. Wanklyn (*Milk Analysis*, by J. Alfred Wanklyn) speaks of the " great difficulty of cream analysis," and says "there is far more difficulty in drying a cream residue than in drying a milk residue," and further says that the whole experimental error, if there is any, " falls on' the determination of the solids not fat, and that any imperfection in the analysis tends to enlarge the solids not fat."

In analyzing cream, the same method should be followed as has already been suggested for the analysis of milk, with three exceptions; in the first portion of the analysis only one, or, at most, two grams of cream should be taken, instead of five cubic centimetres, as in milk analysis; in the second portion, only five grams should be used, instead of ten cubic centimetres, as in milk analysis; and, third, after the fat has been extracted, by agitation with ether and alcohol, the drying of what remains (the casein, sugar, and salts) should be continued until the weight becomes constant. This weight is, of course, that of solids not fat, and, when added to that of the fat which has already been extracted, should tally with the weight of the total solids obtained by drying in the first portion of the analysis. In case these two weights should not tally, the probable explanation is, that in the first portion, the water has not been completely evaporated, for it is very difficult, or almost impossible, if the cream examined is very rich in fat, to obtain a correct weight of the total solids by simple drying in the water-bath.

If condensed milk is to be analyzed, the method should be carried out in the same manner as has already been described, except that in the first part of the analysis only half a gram should be used, and some alcohol mixed with the condensed milk, after the quantity has been weighed, as this seems to facilitate the drying. In the second portion, two grams should be taken instead of ten, as directed when fresh milk is to be analyzed.

3

CHAPTER II.

ANALYSES of human milk, carried out as advised in the previous chapter, seem to show that it never contains the amount of casein commonly supposed, and that in other respects, also, its composition is different from the idea commonly held. Instead of containing two to four per cent. of casein, as is generally supposed, it contains only one per cent. While containing, however, a much smaller amount of casein than cows' milk, there is a larger quantity of sugar and less inorganic matter. The difference between the relative amounts of water and fat is not very great, there being nearly equal quantities of fat and a slightly greater amount of water in human milk ; but the difference is very slight, amounting only to one or two per cent. This may be seen by examining Table VIII, page 77, in which different analyses are placed in parallel columns for comparison, and it shows human milk to be very different from what it is ordinarily supposed to be, and from cows' milk. The analyses of Vernois and Becquerel, which are widely known and much quoted, and of Simon, are almost identical with what cows' milk is now known to be, and therefore they cannot be correct. These analyses are accepted as standard by such well-known authorities as Carpenter, Kirke, Marshall, Edward Smith, Kehrer, and Gorup-Besanez. It is curious how all previous experimenters and writers upon milk agree that human milk contains less casein than does cows'; and yet, when the actual question of the relative composition is arrived at, the mean of Vernois and Becquerel is used as the standard, although their estimate of the quantity of casein is quite as large as the amount granted to be contained in cows' milk.

The observation of the author, therefore, that human milk never contains more than about one per cent. of casein, is an original one ; for, although Henri and Chevallier, and other investigators, long ago arrived at nearly the same analytical results, yet none of them ever enunciated the belief that human milk contains always the small amount of casein, and never three or four per cent., as commonly supposed, thereby denying the correctness of the analyses commonly accepted as standard.

Much has been written of later years, and many experiments have been made, to prove the difference in chemical composition between the casein of cows' and of human milk. Kehrer made an ingenious experiment, separating the coagulum of milk from the serum by forcing the serum through a porous cell by means of an air-pump, and endeavored therefrom to prove that the difference between human and cows' milk lies principally in a difference in the composition and chemical reactions of the two kinds of casein. At the same time, he says the two serums are alike in their reactions, and makes no mention of the great difference in the amounts of casein. Biedert has written a valuable and much quoted article to prove that the caseins of the two milks are essentially, and in their nature, unlike. Both Kehrer and Biedert fail, however, to emphasize the great and cardinal difference—that there is only one-third the quantity of casein in human that there is in cows' milk. Casein is, in its nature, akin to albumen, and the different effects produced when albuminous urines containing different quantities of albumen are boiled and treated with nitric acid are commonly known and understood. If the amount of albumen is small, the coagulation takes place in the form of a mere opalescence of the fluid; the coagula are individually so small that they cannot be seen; whereas, if the amount of albumen be large, the coagulation takes place in heavy white flakes, which are individually easily visible to the naked eye. There is no reason why a parallel explanation of the different coagulability of the two milks should not hold good—that the one contains much less coagulable matter than the other, rather than that some far-away difference should be sought for in the chemical composition of the casein.

While it is true that the great and cardinal difference between human and cows' milk is in the relative proportions of casein contained, it cannot be denied, that there is strong reason to believe that a difference exists (it is impossible, in the present state of our knowledge, to know how great or how little, and of what importance it may be) between the two sorts of casein ; still, this has been given an undue weight, and the great difference in relative quantity, lost sight of. Whatever may finally be proved as to the parallelism or difference of the two sorts of casein, it is indisputable that the casein, which is the coagulable element, is the indigestible portion of cows' milk when used as an article of food for the human infant.

The most important end to be sought for as a result of analysis is to acquire a correct and exact idea of the average composition of the substance analyzed. Therefore, it is necessary to have, before drawing deductions with regard to human milk, or comparing it intelligently with the milk of the lower animals, a scientifically correct understanding of its general average composition. This can only be had by analyzing the milk of a large number of women, under different circumstances and obtained at all sorts of times ; for it is a well-known fact that in cows, the first milk drawn from the animal is much poorer in fat than that which comes last in the milking, or, as it is commonly called, the "strippings." Why this should be so does not seem ever to have been satisfactorily explained, but that it is a fact, and that it holds good with regard to women as well as cows, is beyond dispute. This constitutes one among the various difficulties in obtaining a correct mean of the general composition. The process of analysis which has been recommended,

also, is such a tedious one, taking four to six days
to complete a full proximate analysis, that the time
required to finish a large number would necessarily
be very great. It was suggested that the same or
even a more accurate result would be attained by
taking equal quantities of the milk of many women
and mixing them together, and then analyzing. By
this process a correct idea of the average composition would be acquired, and only one error introduced ; whereas, if separate analyses were made, and
then an average taken, there would, of course, be
the same number of errors introduced as there were
analyses made !

Gerber has recommended that in analyzing human
milk the woman should be made to pass two or three
hours without nursing her child, and then to draw
as much as can be obtained into a vessel, and this,
after careful mixing, used for analytic purposes. He
says that from thirty to two hundred cubic centimetres will usually be obtained, and that both breasts
should be drawn.   This may be good advice, but it is
difficult to follow, for in many women but little milk
can be obtained, either by the use of a breast-pump
or by milking it out with the finger and thumb, even
when the child evidently has no difficulty in obtaining an abundant supply so soon as it is put to the
breast ; and besides, but few women, except paupers,
will submit to have their whole supply taken from
them, for there is then nothing left for the infant, and
it will have to wait several hours, crying, until a fresh
accumulation can take place.   The milk, therefore,

which was used in making the analyses in the accompanying table (Table III) was obtained at all sorts of times, and no attempt was made to draw the

TABLE I.

MILK OF TWENTY-SEVEN WHITE WOMEN IN ALMSHOUSE,
OBTAINED MARCH 23, 1882.

Mother's Age (Years).	Child's Age (Months).	Number of Children Woman had had.	Reaction.
29	3	1	Alkaline.
23	3	2	"
23	5	2	"
22	5	1	"
19	3	2	"
18	9	1	"
18	3	1	"
22	2	1	"
25	12	3	"
27	6½	1	"
23	6	1	"
33	4	6	"
22	5	1	"
25	1	1	"
24	17	1	"
23	1	2	"
22	16	1	"
24	3	1	"
30	6	1	"
33	1	1	"
37	2	7	"
18	14	1	"
34	21	2	"
25	16	1	"
37	2	12	"
38	4	1	"
23	20	1	"

whole supply of milk from the breasts of any one of the women. Where single analyses were made, the usual rule followed was to tell the woman to put

her child to the breast for a minute or two to get
the milk started, and then to draw into a clean bottle
about twenty or twenty-five cubic centimetres. This
gave neither the first milk, which is poor in fat, nor
the rich " strippings," which come last. When the
mixed milk of several women was used, as in the
case of that obtained from the Philadelphia Hospital,
it was taken simply by going into the ward and
making each woman give five cubic centimetres of
milk, and then thoroughly mixing the whole

TABLE II.

MILK OF EIGHT NEGRO WOMEN, OBTAINED MARCH 23, 1882.

Mother's Age (Years).	Child's Age (Months).	Number of Children Woman had had.	Reaction.
20	5	1	Alkaline.
21	12	1	"
43	11	18	"
28	24	2	"
18	1½	2	"
21	2	2	"
22	3	3	"
22	13	2	"

together.   In this way, some of the women had just
nursed their children, some had allowed an hour or
two to pass since the child had been to the breast,
and others were midway between two nursings. This
method would seem, as the women were taken in all
possible stages, to give as fair an average as can
be obtained of the usual composition. Table I
shows the ages of the women, the ages of the infants,
the number of children the women had had, and the

reaction of the milk, in an analysis of the milk of twenty-seven women in the Philadelphia Hospital, and Table II shows the same thing in the analysis made of the milk of eight negro women obtained from the same source. These specimens were kindly furnished by Dr. Fairfield, the resident physician, and were obtained by the permission of Dr. John M. Keating, the visiting physician in charge at the time.

It will be noticed that in every instance (see Table III) in which the reaction was taken with test-paper the milk was alkaline except one, and that was neutral. It is a fact, and one not generally known, that fresh human milk will almost always turn litmus-red paper back to blue again, and cows' milk almost as universally turns litmus-blue paper red. When the milk of the twenty-seven women was obtained at the hospital, Dr. Fairfield got also that of another woman, who was suffering with syphilis, and found it to be markedly acid, and, therefore, it was thrown out as not being a fair sample of healthy milk.

If it be desired to analyze cows' milk, the same process, already so fully described, should be used, and the result will show a larger proportion of inorganic matter (ash), less sugar, and a much greater amount of casein, while the quantities of fat and water will not be found to differ very materially from those existing in human milk. The details of the analysis of cows' milk by this process are much less trying, and it takes less time than when human milk is analyzed; for, as the casein is in

TABLE III.

	No. 1.	No. 2.	No. 3.	No. 4.	No. 5.	No. 6.	No. 7.	No. 8.	No. 9.	No. 10.	Average from Milk of the 43 Women.
	Irish Woman, Lower Class, æt. 30 Years, Child, 15 Mos.	American, Lower Class, æt. 25 Years, Child 6 Mos.	Scotch Woman, Lower Class, æt. 36 Years, Child 10 Mos.	American, Better Class, æt. 30 Years, Child 10 Mos.	American, Better Class.	27 White Women in Almshouse. See Table I.	8 Negro Women in Almshouse. See Table II.	Lower Class.	Lower Class, æt. 26 Years, 3d Child, Child 20 Mos.	Lower Class, æt. 28 Years, 2d Child, æt. 2 Mos.	
	Alkaline.	Alkaline.	Neutral.		Alkaline.			Alkaline.			
Water	87.106	87.695	89.038	83.001	87.306	87.038	87.399	88.489	87.236	88.937	87.163
Fat	4.370	3.682	2.412	9.045	4.498	4.389	3.942	3.211	4.219	2.697	4.283
Casein	1.268	.938	.729	.787	1.083	1.058	1.071	.958	1.155	.912	1.046
Sugar	7.120	7.568	7.704	7.069	6.996	7.417	7.490	7.224	7.292	7.356	7.407
Ash	.136	.117	.117	.098	.117	.098	.098	.118	.098	.098	.101
Total	100.000	100.000	100.000	100.000	100.000	100.000	100.000	100.000	100.000	100.000	100.000
Error	.078 per cent. excess.	no error	.048 per cent. loss.	.049 per cent. loss.	.293 per cent. excess.	.166 per cent. loss.	.157 per cent. loss.	.078 per cent. loss.	.078 per cent. loss.	.215 per cent. loss.	

larger proportion and the sugar less, it does not take nearly so long to dry the sugar residue, in the second portion of the analysis, as when the larger amount of sugar found in human milk has to be dried. The separation of the casein and sugar, also, is more easily effected ; for, as soon as the milk has been shaken with alcohol and ether, the casein being in large quantity (three times as much as in human milk), it at once forms heavy curds, which immediately sink to the bottom of the containing vessel. The casein having formed these large coagula, the dissolved sugar is much more easily poured off into another vessel than when the small, very fine, and light curds of human milk are dealt with ; for, in the latter instance, more of the solid matter necessarily goes over with the sugar, and then the process must be repeated again and again, until at last the solid casein is entirely separated from the dissolved sugar.

The two subjoined analyses constituting Table IV give a fair conception of the average result of analyses of cows' milk, carried out by the method detailed in Chapter I.

TABLE IV.

	Cows' Milk.	Cows' Milk.
Water........................	88.549	87.012
Fat	3.310	4.209
Casein	2.792	3.252
Sugar	4.898	5.000
Ash.........................	.451	.527
Total..................	100.000	100.000
Error	.029 per cent. in excess.	.058 per cent. loss.

TABLE V.

	Eagle Brand Condensed Milk.	Condensed Milk, 1 Teaspoonful (11.233 grams) to 6 Tablespoonfuls (90 c.c.) of Water.
Water.................	27.942	92.673
Fat	10.335	1.095
Casein................	9.522	.868
Sugar	50.861	5.206
Ash...................	1.340	.158
Total............	100.000	100.000
Error..................	.467 per cent. loss.	.009 per cent. loss.

Table V shows analyses of condensed milk and
of a mixture of it with water in about such proportions as should be used if it is to be given as a food
for young infants.

TABLE VI.

	Cream.	Cream.	Creams.	Percentage of Fat in Each.	Creams.	Percentage of Fat in Each.
Water.....	79.122	79.901	No. 1...19.020		No. 12...15.611	
Fat........	13.362	12.470	" 2...17.507		" 13...19.071	
Casein....	2.919	2.846	" 3...13.362		" 14...11.782	
Sugar.....	4.140	4.308	" 4...12.470		" 15...18.519	
Ash........	.457	.475	" 5...17.129		" 16...21.465	
			" 6...16.024		" 17...21.290	
Total....	100.000	100.000	" 7...13.825			
			" 8...14.950		Average percentage from the 17 estimates.	
Error......	.109 per cent. loss.	.039 per cent. in excess.	" 9...18.082			
			" 10...16.502		16.398	
			" 11...12.159			

Table VI shows the results of two full proximate analyses of ordinary cream, and the percentage of fat in seventeen specimens of cream, such as is sold in the city, taken at random from different milk and cream venders. The cream amounts in the full proximate analyses are included in the seventeen fat percentages, being Nos. 3 and 4.

CHAPTER III.

ALTHOUGH many chemists have made analyses
of human milk, and a great variety of divergent results have been attained by different methods, there
has, as yet, been no proof offered of the correctness of any of them. This constitutes an important
missing link in any attempt to place the question
of the composition of milk upon a settled basis ;
and if a method of analysis is ever devised that
will give results which shall be universally accepted,
and stand the test of time, the accuracy and correctness of the method must be susceptible of proof
—simple, scientific, and incontrovertible proof. To
prove the correctness of the analyses already given,
will be the object of this chapter.

No one disputes that in ether, chemists have a
perfect solvent for fat, which, when properly applied
in milk analysis, extracts it all. The fat, when separated, can be seen, and the eye tells positively that
it is fat.

With regard to the water, it is equally certain
that by the evaporation process its amount can be
accurately estimated. This statement is made with
the knowledge that there may be with the water
some slight traces of other fluids—alcohol, for in-

stance, and, perhaps other volatile liquids; but these must be in such minute quantity that they need not be taken into consideration; and, for the present, the liquid portion of milk may be spoken of as the water. It is equally certain that in incineration, properly performed, there exists an easy and correct method of determining the amount of inorganic matter. In the future, of course, there may be perfected some way of estimating the salts in milk, by extracting from the liquid milk, or from the solid residue left after evaporation; and this may show them to exist in larger quantity than the present method of incineration leads to believe; but the possible error introduced in this way must be very small, and does not invalidate the general facts stated.

That the existing estimates of the water, fat, and inorganic matter are correct, is further proved by the fact that there is no difference of opinion in regard to their amounts. Examination of the analyses of different chemists shows an almost exact uniformity of conclusion with regard to the relative quantities of the above-mentioned substances.

When the estimates of the casein and sugar, however, are considered, the widest divergence of view is discovered in the conclusions as to the amounts existing in human milk. In regard to cows' milk, chemists all arrive at nearly uniform conclusions. The casein in human milk is estimated by Dolan and Wood, in one of their analyses, at 7.005 per cent.; Vernois and Becquerel give it as 3.924 per

TABLE VII.

	Vernois and Becquerel.	Simon.	Henri and Chevallier.	Dolan and Wood.	Haidlen.	L'Héritier.	Doyère.	Clemm.	Tidy.	Meigs.	Payen.	Quevenne.	Regnault.
Casein..	3.924	3.43	1.52	7.005	3.1	1.30	.85	3.533	3.533	1.046	.215	1.05	3.9
Sugar...	4.364	4.82	6.50	1.921	4.3	7.80	7.31	4.118	4.624	7.407	8.805	7.31	4.9
Total...	8.288	8.25	8.02	8.926	7.4	9.10	8.16	7.651	8.157	8.453	9.020	8.36	8.8

The estimates of Haidlen, L'Héritier, Doyère, and Clemm are taken from a table in the *Physiologische Chemie* of Gorup-Besanez; those of Vernois and Becquerel, Payen and Regnault, are taken from one in the *Traité de Chimie Pathologique*, par Becquerel et Rodier; but the others are from the original sources. A complete estimate of all the constituents is not attempted in the analysis of Quevenne; and under the head which is called casein in the table is included albumen (matière albumineuse précipitée par l'alcool); under that of sugar are included, also, extractive matters (lactine et matières extractives).

cent., and Henri and Chevallier as 1.52 per cent., while the original analyses already quoted seem to show that there is about 1 per cent. Now, the fact is a striking one, that if, in any of these analyses, the sugar and casein amounts be added together, the sums are found to be in each instance nearly the same. Table VII shows this to be the case.

The table also shows that in each instance where the casein amount is large, the sugar is small, and *vice versâ*—that where the casein amount is small, that of sugar is large.

It has been already said that, as regards the analysis of human milk, all observers are agreed as to the proportions of the water, fat, and ash ; it is now further evident, from the table, that all agree as to the quantities of casein and sugar taken collectively, and that only when the separation of the two is attempted does there exist any difference of opinion. The separation of the casein from the sugar, therefore, is the difficult part of milk analysis, for in regard to this alone is there any difference of opinion. In this portion of milk analysis, then, is reached the stumbling-block, and it alone requires any explanation, for the rest is universally conceded, and cannot therefore but be considered as already placed upon a scientifically exact basis.

There are but two possible explanations of the different results arrived at by various investigators ; one, that human milk is as variable a substance in regard to the amounts of casein and sugar contained

4

as the different analyses would lead to believe ; and
the other, that the methods of the majority of chemists have been faulty and their conclusions incorrect.
That the second of these·two explanations is the
correct one, does not admit of doubt.   Wanklyn
says that cows' milk is a substance exhibiting great
uniformity of composition, and what he says of
cows' milk is also probably true of human milk.
There is no reason to expect that it would vary so
much in regard to the proportions of casein and
sugar, when cows' milk exhibits such uniformity of
composition in these respects.   It may, by analogy,
be fairly argued that human milk is very unlikely
to be so variable as published analyses would seem
to show.   The proof of this, however, lies in showing, by examination of a large number of specimens, that human milk always contains a large
amount of sugar (say seven per cent.) and therefore
by exclusion, it cannot contain the great amount of
casein it is usually credited with, for all observers
agree as to the sum of the amounts of the two substances.

The existence of this large amount of sugar in human milk, it was attempted to demonstrate by exper-
imenting as to how much could be obtained in the
crystalline form from any fixed quantity, and then,
by applying the same process to cows' milk, to find
out whether an equal or, as should be the case if
the already published original analyses are correct,
only a less quantity of sugar will take the crystalline form.

An experiment was made as follows : 10 c.c. of human milk, which had already, by the process described, been found to contain 7.224 per cent. of sugar was, as usual, agitated with ether and alcohol, and the fat removed. After the removal of the fat the remaining portion was carefully washed into a dish, and in the water-bath, at a temperature of 70° to 80° C., evaporated until only about 10 c.c. of fluid remained ; upon this was poured a mixture of 25 c.c. of water with 25 c.c. of alcohol, and the whole allowed to stand over night. By morning a precipitate had formed and settled to the bottom of the vessel ; this was thrown upon a filter and washed with a mixture of equal parts of boiling alcohol and water. The filtrate was again reduced in the water-bath, at a temperature of 70° to 80° C., to about 10 c.c., and then 75 c.c. of absolute alcohol added. This caused again the formation of a slight precipitate, which was allowed to thoroughly settle to the bottom, when the perfectly clear fluid above was poured off into a dish, care being taken that none of the precipitate passed over with the clear fluid. This liquid was allowed to evaporate, without heat, in an open dish of known weight, and there remained, finally, only crystalline milk-sugar, with a very minute amount of the inorganic material. The 10 c.c. of milk thus treated yielded 659 milligrammes of sugar dry at 100° C. This milk had been previously ascertained to contain 738 milligrammes of sugar to each 10 c.c., which made its percentage of sugar 7.224, as already stated.

That all the sugar which existed in the 10 c.c. of milk was not obtained (nor was such a thing attempted), is proved by the fact that if a concentrated solution of milk-sugar in water is treated with an excess of alcohol, the precipitation of a considerable quantity of sugar takes place ; and this occurs in proportion as the original sugar solution is concentrated, and the amount of alcohol added large. This fact, which is easily demonstrated by making a solution of crystalline milk-sugar in water and then treating with alcohol, of course occurred in the above-described process, some of the sugar falling with the casein when alcohol was added, as was done twice ; and, therefore, the clear fluid poured off from the precipitate did not contain all the sugar, but some remained behind in the solid form with the casein.

The figures given are sufficiently nearly parallel to prove the point, for, by the method of crystallization described, it was not expected that all the sugar present would be obtained. The effort was made merely to obtain it pure, and in sufficient quantity to prove that the sugar existed in the milk in the large quantity shown by the analysis, and therefore necessarily, by exclusion, the existence of only the small amount of casein. The demonstration thus obtained seems incontrovertible, for when the existence of the large amount of sugar is shown, it follows as a necessary corollary that there can be only the small amount of casein.

As a means of further proving that the sugar obtained by crystallization, as described, was entirely free from any traces of casein, it was tested by Mr. J. K. Hecker, the apothecary of the Pennsylvania Hospital, by the Nessler test described by Wanklyn and Chapman (*Water Analysis*, by J. Alfred Wanklyn and Ernest Theopron Chapman, London, 1876, p. 25). This test decomposes the casein and forms ammonia from the nitrogen. When the crystalline sugar was subjected to its action, it showed it to be practically free from casein.

Cows' milk, when subjected to the same process of precipitation of the casein by alcohol, after the removal of the fat, yielded only about four or five per cent. of crystalline sugar. The manipulations were not carried out with the same exactitude as when human milk was examined, for there is no dispute as to the amount of sugar in cows' milk; the experiment was therefore made merely to afford confirmatory evidence of what was shown by that upon the human milk. For if only a little more than four per cent. of sugar existed in human milk, as is claimed by Vernois and Becquerel, and others, and this being the quantity universally conceded to exist in cows' milk, then, both being subjected to the action of the same reagents, the same amount only of crystalline sugar should be yielded. This, however, was not the case.

One of the strongest proofs of the correctness of the estimates of fat in milk is afforded by the fact that after it has been separated, it can be seen, and the eye tells that it is fat. When sugar is crystallized, can be seen and felt, and examined with the microscope or a magnifying-glass; the characteristically shaped crystals of milk-sugar are seen, and the fact that it is sugar, and nothing else, becomes self-evident.

To test still further the accuracy of the method described, a specimen of human milk was analyzed and found to contain the different proximate constituents in about the usual quantities. There were then separated from a further portion of the milk, taken at the same time and under exactly parallel circumstances, fresh portions of the casein and sugar, which were given to Mr. Hecker to test their purity—the sugar to be subjected to the Nessler test, to discover if it contained any casein, and the casein to be subjected to the action of Fehling's test, to find whether or not it was free from all traces of sugar. The casein entirely failed to produce any effect upon the copper solution, thus showing that it was free from sugar, while, if a small portion of the sugar was added to the solution, the characteristic reduction of the copper at once took place. When the sugar was subjected to the Nessler test, .05 gram being introduced into the retort when the decomposing materials were ready, it almost entirely failed to react, showing no more change than would be accounted for by the distilled water which had been used to prepare the reagents. This distilled water must have contained traces of organic matter, for when it was subjected to the test it showed slight traces of ammonia. The test is so delicate, that it is only by the greatest care and nicety in preparing the materials that they can be had perfectly free from all nitrogenized materials. The conclusion was that the sugars—both that prepared by the ordinary process advised for analytic purposes, and that obtained by crystallization—were, practically speaking, free from casein.

One of the strongest corroborative evidences of the correctness of the low estimate of the casein in human milk is that when cream, milk, water, limewater, and milk-sugar are mixed together in proportions presently to be described, the resulting mixture is, in its appearance, taste, and reactions, strikingly like human milk ; much more so than any of the other mixtures recommended as infant foods. This mixture is known to contain fat, casein, milk-sugar, and water in the same proportions as the analyses of the author seem to show that they exist in human milk, for it is fair to assume as known quantities the proportions of the various constituents in cows' milk and cream, and these being known, it is easy, by arithmetical process, to construct a mixture which shall contain the various constituents in any desired amounts. That this mixture should react, when subjected to the same process of analysis that has been recommended for human milk in an almost exactly similar manner, is certainly very striking, and tends, at least, to show that the liquids are nearly identical.

If, then, it has been shown that human milk contains approximately 87.1 per cent. of water, 4.2 per cent. of fat, 7.4 per cent. of sugar, and 0.1 per cent. of inorganic matter, the proof that it contains, not three or four per cent. of casein, as is commonly taught, but only about one per cent., is complete.

CHAPTER IV.

THE best known analyses of human milk are those of Vernois and Becquerel, and their results have been accepted as standard by most writers upon physiology and foods. A full account of their methods and results is contained in the *Traité de Chimie Pathologique*, par Becquerel et Rodier, Paris, 1854, at page 393. The original article will be found in the *Ann. d'hyg.*, p. 257. In attempting a criticism of the methods pursued, that of Vernois and Becquerel will first be discussed, as their mean has been so widely quoted and is the result of eighty-nine analyses of human milk made by them. In pursuing their method, the milk to be analyzed was divided into two equal portions; from the first they estimated, in the usual manner, the amount of water by evaporation, the total solids by the residue left, the fat by extracting with ether from the dried residue, and the inorganic matter (ash) by inciner-ation; so far, therefore, their results coincide accu-rately with those of almost all other authorities. When, however, the second portion of the analysis—the separation of the casein and sugar—is reached, they direct that thirty grams of milk be taken and curdled by heating to the boiling-point, after adding

49

one or two drops of rennet and a few drops of acetic acid. This is filtered, and the clear filtrate, they say, constitutes the serum, which consists of the sugar, extractive matters, and soluble salts. The amount of sugar in this serum was then estimated by means of the "polarimètre."* This gives, they say, the exact quantity of sugar contained in the thirty grams. If this process is carried out, it is found that the milk does curdle, to be sure, but the coagulum, which contains much the larger part of the fat (none of which has been previously removed) as well as the casein, is of such a consistency that the moment it is thrown upon a filter it seems to fill all the pores of the paper, and nearly twenty-four hours are required to complete the filtration process. This, of course, makes it quite impossible to wash the residue left upon the filter, for if the attempt is made to pass any water through the mass of coagulum upon the paper, twenty-four hours more would be required, and during that time fermentation would have occurred to such an extent as to entirely vitiate the results acquired. Fermentation is very apt to have begun, even when no attempt at washing is made, before the liquid has all drained through the paper, and must, to some slight extent, therefore, vitiate the accuracy of the results. Hav-

---

* " Pour connaître la quantité de sucre, on soumet le sérum au polarimètre, et en étudiant le degré de déviation du rayon polarisé et recherchant sur une table constituée d' avance, sa déviation, on a la quantité exacte du sucre de lait contenue dans 1000 grammes de sérum du lait."

ing by these processes obtained the weights of the
sugar, fat, etc., that of the casein is estimated by
difference.

The fallacy of this process is, that during the long
time which is required to effect the separation of
the coagulum from the matters remaining in solution, by passing the latter through a filter-paper, a
considerable portion of sugar crystallizes upon the
paper, more is entangled in the coagulum, which, as
has already been said, it is impossible to wash; and
thus the serum which is finally obtained, does not
contain all the sugar, quite a large portion of which
has remained with the casein upon the filter, and is,
therefore, classed with it as casein. Further, the
expediency of estimating by difference any element
in making an analysis of an organic substance is
very doubtful, as being likely to lead to error. If
by any means it can be effected, each element
should be individually separated, so that it may be
seen and felt, and the fact of its being the substance
supposed, thoroughly established by testing. The
use of so large an amount of milk as thirty grams
for evaporation and estimation of the total solids
and water is also inadvisable. Simon* opens his
article upon milk by saying, " Perfectly fresh milk
has always a decidedly alkaline reaction, and it
retains this property for a longer or shorter time :
the milk of women retains its alkaline reaction
longer than that of cows, etc." That this is not

---

* *Animal Chemistry*, *etc.*, by Dr. J. Franz Simon. Sydenham
Society Translation.

true of cows' milk, the author has proved by testing
with litmus paper the milk of about thirty healthy
cows, one evening, at a locally famous dairy farm.
The milk was drawn directly into a vessel from the
teat and immediately tested, and in almost every
instance it distinctly reddened the test-paper. In
one or two cases only the color of the paper
remained unchanged, and further testing with
turmeric paper yielded also negative results, showing
that the milk was neutral in reaction; but in no
single instance was there the slightest evidence of
alkalinity. Simon estimates the water and total
solids, as usual, by evaporation, and then extracts
the fat from the dried residue with boiling ether.
The remaining portion is pulverized and digested
with a little boiling water, and the solution evaporated at a gentle temperature to the consistence of
a thin syrup, when it is treated with ten or twelve
times its volume of alcohol of 0.85 per cent., which
precipitates the casein, and with it, as he justly
observes, some of the sugar. This manipulation is
repeated once or oftener, and, finally, the casein
dried. Simon himself was not well satisfied with
the results thus obtained, for he says : " This analysis of milk does not yield, as Berzelius justly
observes, any very accurate results, etc."

The fallacy of this method is caused by the fact
that milk-sugar is entirely insoluble in absolute alcohol, and only can be dissolved in alcohol as it
becomes dilute, and further, because, as Simon himself says, if a concentrated solution of milk-sugar

in water is treated with alcohol, a precipitation of the sugar is caused. This fact renders it impossible to know, if the method of Simon is pursued, when all the sugar is removed from the precipitated casein.

The original article of Chevallier and O. Henri has not been accessible to the author, but an account of their method and results is given by Simon.* They precipitated the casein with acetic acid and estimated the sugar by evaporation of the fluid portion, and then by incineration determined its amount, the loss in burning being set down as the amount of sugar. Simon does not say how the separation of the fluid portion from the precipitate was effected, but it must probably have been by filtration; and this, if true, would account for the fact that their estimate of casein is slightly too high. If fluid milk is curdled with acetic acid, and then an attempt made to filter off the fluid portion, it will be found, as has already been said, that the coagulum, which consists almost wholly of fat and casein, is of such a consistence that when it is put upon a filter-paper it soon stops the pores of the paper, so that filtration takes place only very slowly. As evaporation goes on to a considerable degree, the portion of the filter-paper above the liquid is by capillary attraction kept constantly soaked with the solution of sugar, and gradually a good deal of sugar is left upon the upper portion of the paper,

---

* *Loc. cit.*

and some also is entangled in the coagulum. All this sugar is, in the final calculation, classed with the casein. The error, however, thus introduced is small when compared with that of other methods, and consequently the analysis of Chevallier and Henri is more nearly correct than any heretofore published. Their analysis is the one which has been accepted by Lethby* as his standard of the composition of human milk.

It is with great hesitation that a criticism of the process of analysis of Wanklyn† is approached. The method suggested by him is the best, and offers more nearly accurate results than any other as yet published, and has, so far as the analysis of cows' milk is concerned, been a great step in advance in the effort to arrive at an exact knowledge of the composition of milk. That almost all chemical processes are susceptible of improvement is, however, a fact that is indisputable, and that suggested by the author, although it is believed to be an advance upon the old methods, will, in its turn also, doubtless be cast aside for some other one still more easy, rapid, and accurate. Wanklyn, in his treatise, confines himself to the consideration of cows' milk, but the fault that may be found with it as a means for the examination of cows' milk also holds good when it is applied to human milk. His method of extracting the fat from the dried residue with ether is the same as has been pursued by others, and it

---

* *On Food, etc.*, by H. Lethby.   London, 1870.
† *Milk Analysis*, by J. Alfred Wanklyn.

gives, if carefully carried out, fairly accurate results, but is much more tedious and troublesome than the method suggested by the author; besides which, if the fat is extracted from the liquid milk and the remainder then dried, it renders much more easy the subsequent separation of the casein and sugar, and there is less risk of loss, as the amount of necessary handling is much reduced. Wanklyn says of the separation of the casein and sugar, that it should be effected " by extracting with strong alcohol, and ultimately adding a little boiling water, so as in effect to extract with very weak hot alcohol, the milk-sugar, and the soluble part of the ash, *i. e.*, the chlorides, will pass into solution." The sugar is estimated by evaporating to dryness and then incinerating, the loss in burning being the weight of the sugar. The separation of the solution from the undissolved casein is effected by filtration. This method is open to criticism, for two reasons. First, because milk-sugar is almost totally insoluble in strong alcohol, and therefore alcohol is perfectly useless in dissolving out the sugar from the residue, unless it is used because its presence is supposed to prevent the casein going into solution with the sugar; for the sugar is dissolved, not by alcohol but by the water with which it is diluted. It will be found, also, that if it is attempted to dissolve milk-sugar in a liquid containing any but a very small amount of alcohol, the solution will take place only very slowly; and this might easily be anticipated, when it is recollected that alcohol will cause milk-sugar to precipitate when it is mixed with a watery solution of the sugar. This being so, the attempt to separate the casein and sugar with dilute alcohol is very likely to cause error by some of the sugar remaining behind undissolved with the casein. Second, as the final separation of the solution from the solid residue is directed to be effected by filtration, the sources of error already mentioned in connection with the observations upon the method of Chevallier and Henri are liable to be fallen into; and further, all paper filters will allow quite a considerable portion of the casein which has coagulated in fine particles to pass through. This observation is confirmed by one recently made by Dr. F. P. Henry,* that if blood was thrown upon an ordinary filter-paper, even when a very small quantity was used, about one-third of the red corpuscles passed through and were found in the filtrate. This was established by a careful use of the hæmacytometer, the number of corpuscles being counted both before and after filtration, when it was found that one-third of the number originally present had passed through the paper. If filter-paper will allow blood corpuscles to pass through its meshes, it surely cannot be depended upon to prevent the passage of the finer particles of coagulated casein.

The possible error involved in following the method of Wanklyn is, after all however, very small, and infinitely less than that introduced by

* *Archives of Medicine*, October, 1882. A Contribution to the Study of Anæmia.

most other analysts, and it amounts merely to causing a slightly too large estimate of the casein at the expense of the sugar.

Many analysts of milk have estimated the amount of sugar by the copper test, using Fehling's solution. The results obtained in this way by different investigators are so various that it is impossible they can all be correct, and a large part of the divergent conclusions attained must be set down to error. It would be absurd at this day to attempt to cast any doubt upon the value of the copper test, both as a means of qualitative and quantitative estimation of sugar ; but when it is introduced into new fields, and there is no means of correcting the results acquired, it alone having to be depended upon to decide the amount of one constituent, and another which is in intimate admixture or solution being estimated by difference, the results should be scrutinized with great care and only accepted with extreme caution. When, however, different analyses of human milk are examined, the estimates of the sugar and casein—for, as has already (pp. 39-41) been so carefully shown, it is upon the amounts of these two elements alone that any difference of opinion exists—arrived at even by the same author in different analyses, are so widely apart that, if the truth of Wanklyn's observation as to the uniformity of composition of cows' milk applies at all to human milk, all cannot be correct. Dolan and Wood* give thir-

---

* *The Practitioner* for February, March, April, and May, 1882. Article upon Human Milk.

teen original analyses of human milk, and in one
they set down the amount of casein at 7.005 per
cent. and that of sugar 1.921 per cent., in another
the casein is 3.603 per cent. and sugar 4.507 per
cent.

In these analyses the sugar amount is taken by
the use of the copper test, and then the casein estimated by difference. If the estimates are correct,
and milk is really so variable a substance as they
would seem to prove, analysis, as a means of understanding its composition and of helping toward a
conclusion as to how best to artificially feed infants,
had better be abandoned ; for it will be quite impossible ever to make a food like a substance, different
specimens of which are more unlike than the milks
even of any two of the lower animals are represented
to be. The copper test is so delicate, and such
various directions are given as to the exact manner
for using it, that, as such different estimates of the
amount of sugar in a substance which all the other
facts would seem to show to be very uniform in composition, it is fair to conclude that the explanation
of the difference is caused by error. It is certainly a
very difficult thing, when dealing with unknown
quantities of milk-sugar (lactose), to convert it all
into glucose, as must first be done, and then by the
Fehling's solution to arrive at an exact knowledge
of the amount in the solution examined ; so difficult
is it, that many supposed competent chemists have
been led into serious error in the attempt, and have
published results which will not bear the test of

searching examination. Therefore, if an exact comprehension of the composition of human milk is to be attained, the first step must be to throw out all analyses in which the sugar was estimated by the copper test and the casein thence by difference. The copper test seems to give reliable and fairly exact results when known quantities of sugar are dealt with, as is the case in examining cows' milk, for so many analyses have been already made that it is known beforehand very nearly how much sugar will be found.

There have been lately published two papers by Dr. Albert R. Leeds,* giving the results of a large number of analyses made by the Gerber Ritthausen's method. The results attained by Dr. Leeds have been fully discussed, and an attempt to show their fallaciousness made, by the author in a paper read before the College of Physicians, which will appear in the *Transactions of the College of Physicians of Philadelphia*, 3d Series, Vol. VIII. It is not necessary to go fully into the subject here, for the process is like many of the older ones, except that sulphate of copper and caustic potash are used to precipitate the casein in the form of an albuminate of copper.

Enough has now been said about the previous methods of analysis to show that there is certainly good ground for questioning their accuracy, if it has not been shown that they are all to a greater or less degree inexact; and the effort has been made

---

* *Transactions of the College of Physicians of Philadelphia*, 3d Series, Vols. VI and VII, 1883 and 1884.

to prove that the method suggested by the author is exact, or, at any rate, more nearly so than any hitherto published.   Unless, then, it can be shown that the reasoning in the previous chapter does not constitute proof, the statements made with regard to the amounts of casein and sugar which exist in human milk have been demonstrated.   Nothing, therefore, will be said about the various other methods of analysis, for they are but modifications of those which have already been criticised.

CHAPTER V.

In the endeavor to find a food which shall be the best for infants who have to be hand-fed, there are two considerations, either of which might be selected as a basis from which to start. In the first place, the desired goal might be attained by making trial of all sorts of foods, and these being put to the test of experience, the good would be retained and the bad gradually weeded out, until, at last, perhaps the most suitable would be found and slowly introduced. On the other hand, the desired end might be attained by trying to produce a food which should be, as nearly as possible, like what nature has provided for the infant. Many trials have been made in the past by both these methods, but to the second one justice has never been done; for, if the conclusions already detailed are correct, a proper understanding of the composition of human milk, from which to start, has been wanting.

A clear understanding being now had of its proximate constituents, and the proportions in which they exist, it is possible more intelligently to set about finding how the same elements may be had, and mixed together to make an artificial food like human milk. Cows' milk is almost universally the basis of the foods used, in this country at least.

The artificial food which will presently be recommended is the outcome of a study of the subject
from both of the stand-points suggested, and its
advantages are demonstrable. Upon theoretical
grounds, it is what a food for infants should be ;
for analysis of human milk and cows' milk has
shown what their composition is, and in the artificial food the elements have been introduced in the
same proportions as they exist in human milk.
Experience has for many years past been tending
in the direction of proving such a food to be what
is needed ; for, while almost innumerable manufactured infant foods of every variety have been introduced, and have often, for a time, been thought all
that could be desired, they have all, one · after
another, fallen into disuse and been forgotten ; but
the use of cows' milk continues to hold its own, and
in civilized countries is employed ten times more
than all the manufactured foods together. The
question however, remains, of how to use it, and
the various methods suggested have been almost as
numerous as the physicians who have advised
them. For a long time the great majority of
writers upon infant diseases and diet have recommended that cows' milk should be diluted before
giving it to young infants; and this, they agree, is
because it contains too much casein, which causes
a curd that only infants of the strongest digestion
can with safety assimilate.

Although it is true that the majority of authorities advise that cows' milk should be diluted, still,

there have always been those who used it undiluted. Parrot* says, " in my opinion, it is always best to give the milk pure."

Jacobi † disapproves of the use of cream in any form, saying : " It is almost certain that we give too much fat; it is scarcely ever probable that there is too little. Therefore, the addition of cream is rep-rehensible, no matter in what shape." He states (page 110) that human milk contains less fat than cows' milk, but does not say upon what analyses he bases this conclusion. He seems to found his ob-jection to the use of cream upon the fact that Wegscheider found that the " fats are not completely absorbed ; one part leaves the intestine in a saponi-fied condition ; a second part, as free, fatty acid ; a third, as fat in an unchanged condition.

" Where no food is given but mother's milk, which contains fat in proportionately smaller quan-tities than cows' milk, and finely suspended and easily absorbed, a good deal of fat is eliminated."

It seems scarcely wise, upon such purely theoret-ical grounds, to condemn the use of cream, particu-larly when the experience of many physicians has been that they were able to feed successfully upon cream, or cream mixtures, children they were unable to manage in any other way. Surely, Dr.

---

* *Clinique des Nouveau-Nés, L' Athrepsie*, par J. Parrot. Paris, 1877, page 437.

† *Hygiene and Public Health*, edited by Albert H. Buck. New York, 1879, Vol. I, p. 112.

Jacobi would not condemn the use of human milk
because fat may be found in the stools!

The weight of testimony that cows' milk contains
much more casein than human milk, is so great that
it is astonishing how almost universally the analyses
of human milk of Vernois and Becquerel, and of
those who have arrived at like conclusions, have
been accepted and given credence, in despite of the
fact that the evidence of the senses of every one
who has examined into the matter is diametrically
opposed to such an acceptance.   Although, as
already said, the weight of authority has long been
in favor of the use of diluted milk, still, there have
always been those who recommended it to be used
pure.   Of later years more and more has been said
and written upon the advantages to be derived from
the use of cream, or diluted cream.   Dr. J. Forsyth
Meigs, who was a well-known authority upon the
complaints of children, used with great success a
mixture of equal parts of milk, cream, lime-water,
and a weak arrowroot-water, with a little sugar.
Cream mixed with whey, to increase the sugar and
lessen the amount of casein, has been recommended.
Biedert (Virchow's *Archiv*, Band 60, 1874) has
written an article, and concludes that the best-food
is cream and water, one part to four, with 15 grams
of milk-sugar to the half litre of the mixture, the
strength of this to be gradually increased.   Biedert
made many experiments comparing the relative
coagulability of human and cows' milk, and again
the digestibility of the coagulum ; as can therefore

be presupposed, his experiments turned mainly upon the two kinds of casein and their differences. He concludes that " there are two important points in which human and cows' milk are unlike: first, in the different amounts of casein contained; and second, in the absolute chemical difference of the two sorts of casein. The first of these consider-ations would be of little importance, however, if the analyses which place the average of casein in human milk at 4 per cent. are correct; its importance, on the other hand, would be very great if it usually contains—as I, in agreement with Vierordt's view, believe—only from 2 to 2½ per cent. I think many further analyses are necessary to establish absolutely this point. Even if this view is accepted, however, dilution of cows' milk with equal or more parts of water is not sufficient to remove the differences. It is well known that such a dilution does not remove all the disadvantages which arise in the use of cows' milk, and my clinical experience has taught me that even dilution with two parts of water does not attain the desired end; and the explanation of this positive irremovable difference is to be found in the impor-tant chemical differences which exist, the casein of cows' milk coagulating so much more easily, and the coagulum being so much more firm than is the case with the casein of human milk; and, on the other hand, the coagulum being so much more difficult of solution or digestion.

" Until we succeed in actually making the casein of cows' milk identical with that of human milk, it will be necessary to give infants only so much of it as they can digest (no matter how great the necessary dilution may be), and to make up to them with carbo-hydrates (fat and milk-sugar) the lack of albuminates in the food." He further says : "After numerous experiments, I have come to the conclusion that the amount of cow casein which an infant's food should contain is 1 per cent. The fat and sugar in cows' milk appear to be as easily digested, and in no wise different from those contained in human milk. If, therefore, one-eighth of a litre of sweet cream (which, according to Hoppe, contains 9½ per cent. of fat, 3 per cent. of sugar, and 4 per cent. of casein) is diluted with three-eighths of a litre of water, which has been previously boiled, and milk-sugar is added in the proportion of 15 grams to the half litre, the desired cream mixture is produced, and contains 1 per cent. of casein, 2.4 per cent. of fat, and 3.6 per cent. of milk-sugar, which will be found, under all circumstances, to be well borne, and is a sufficiently nourishing food." The greatest part of Biedert's admirable article consists of a detail of experiments made of treating cows' and human milk, and the caseins obtained from both sorts, with a variety of reagents, and observing the different relative effects produced. His conclusion is that "the pure casein of human milk is, in both its physical and chemical nature, different from that of cows' milk." The casein of cows' milk, when isolated, has always an acid reaction, while, on the contrary, that obtained from human milk is always alkaline. If human casein is treated in a certain way with acid, there is produced an "acid modification of human casein," which has many points of resemblance with ordinary cow casein; on the other hand, by treating cow casein with alkali, a substance is produced which shows, with many reagents, identically the same changes that are, by like treatment, produced in human milk. After careful examination of these two substances, however, Biedert concludes that "cow casein treated with alkali is, in many respects, much more like human casein than the original cow casein; yet it always shows unmistakable differences." Although he makes a strong case, and there are many reasons in favor of accepting his conclusions, yet, in the present state of knowledge of casein, the difference cannot be considered as absolutely demonstrated.

There are objections to such a belief: it has been already shown that human milk contains only one-third the amount of casein that exists in cows' milk; and there is a further important difference, which Biedert also appreciates, that human milk is always alkaline, while, on the contrary, cows' milk is acid. A coagulum, therefore, produced in a solution which is relatively so concentrated as is the case in cows' milk, and further, in a fluid which is acid in reaction, is a very much denser and larger one than can be had from the relatively weak solution in human milk; and it is quite possible, therefore, that the difference may be owing to the different degrees of concentration, and the difference of the fluid media in which the casein is held; it cannot, therefore, yet be conceded that Biedert has absolutely demonstrated that the two caseins are chemically and physically different, although he has brought many strong arguments to bear. It is impossible to decide with certainty about casein in all its relations, while as yet it is not even known whether it is a simple or compound substance.

Its solubility or insolubility after it has once been precipitated, depends, in great part, upon how the original coagulation was effected, and whether or not it was thoroughly dried. If casein is once thoroughly dried for a good many hours at 100° C., it becomes absolutely insoluble in water, and will not dissolve even in a strong solution of caustic soda. Lehman (*Physiological Chemistry*, Cavendish Society Translation, Vol. I, p. 378) says: " I believe that the jelly-like coagula of women's milk are more dependent on the alkaline state of the fluid than on any peculiarity in the casein; at all events, I have found that women's milk, when acid, yields a much thicker coagulum than when alkaline, and cows' milk, when alkaline, a much looser coagulum than when acid—facts of the highest interest and value in relation to dietetics.''

Whatever may finally be decided about casein— whether those of cows' and human milk are as different as Biedert believes he has proved, or whether they are nearly alike, the difference being merely that the quantities are not the same and the containing fluid media different—what most concerns the subject in hand is the relatively small quantity that exists in human milk; for it shows conclusively that in a food for infants, the amount of casein in cows' milk must, by some means, be reduced to equal the amount in human milk. The correct conclusion of Biedert, that not more than one per cent. of cow casein should be present in a food for infants, is the more surprising as he arrives at the opinion from a totally different reason from the true one, that human milk contains only one per cent.

Although Biedert's conclusions are very instructive, as he arrives at them from clinical experience, and surprisingly correct in many respects, he goes astray in assuming an incorrect standard of the average composition of cream. The estimate of Hoppe, which he assumes to be correct, places the amount of casein too high; for, as may be seen by a reference to Tables IV and VI, cows' milk and cream do not contain more casein than sugar. The usual estimates rate the casein too high, at the expense of the sugar. This being the case, and Biedert reckoning the composition of his cream mixture from an incorrect standard, and not from any analysis, either of the cream or the mixture itself, as should have been done, places his fat amount too low, as only a very poor cream is as weak in fat as his standard rates it. A mixture made as he directs, is far weaker in sugar than human milk, and therefore, although perhaps proper for temporary use in cases of indigestion, cannot be accepted as a standard of what an infant food should be ; and it entirely fails to accomplish what he says should be done—make up to the infant by an excess of carbo-hydrates the lack of albuminates which exists in the food—for it only contains about half as much sugar as exists in human milk.

In a later work than that which has already been so extensively quoted by Biedert,* he states that the differences between the coagula produced by rennet in cows' and woman's milk are as follows : " first, the different percentages of casein ; second, the different menstrua, especially in regard to the amount of free alkali ; third, in the absolute chemical differences between the two sorts of casein." He finds fault with the statement that human milk contains only about one per cent. of casein, and the suggestion that in this, the great difference in the amounts of casein, lies the most important difference between human and cows' milk, and not in any chemical difference between the two kinds of casein, which is not even as yet positively proved, although Dr. Biedert thinks it has been. Biedert is in error when he says the Nessler's reagent will not act upon unaltered casein, but will act only after it has been converted into ammonia. He reiterates his former statement that the best food for new-born infants is his cream mixture with milk-sugar (cream, 125 grams ; water, which has been boiled, 375, and milk-sugar, 15).

---

* *Untersuchungen über die Chemischen Unterschiede der Menschen und Kuhmilch*, von Dr. Ph. Biedert, Stuttgart, 1884, pages 2, 48, 60, and 61.

All these facts show that the tendency has been constantly toward the truth, and that physicians have been learning empirically for what reasons cows' milk has failed as an infant food, and how the difficulties which its use entailed were to be overcome. The use of cream has been advised; cream and whey; diluted milk; diluted milk with milk-sugar; cream, milk, lime-water, and arrowroot-water; and finally comes Biedert's cream mixture, and he arrives more nearly at the true solution of the difficulty than any of the others, but still falls wide of the mark, from want of a precise knowledge of the composition of human milk, and of cows' milk and cream.

Investigators have thus, year by year and step by step, been approaching the desired goal, and it needed but a touch for light to be let in upon the whole subject. Many hours and much careful and patient labor have been expended upon investigations in this field, and no single worker could have done his part without having before him the results of the labors of his predecessors to guide him a long way in the field, and give him easily the knowledge which would enable him, after much toil and trouble, to advance one little step more toward what was previously unknown. Thus, no individual investigator, no matter how important the advance in knowledge he may have made, should assume too large a share of credit; for it can be but a very small part of the great whole, and would be value-less but for the rest, into which it fits, and completes that which would otherwise be useless.

The necessary data being now at hand, it is com-
paratively easy to construct a food which shall at
least be more nearly what is needed than any previous one.   In making such a food there are two
matters to be considered : the proximate constituents
must be in the same relative proportions as they
are found in human milk, and they must be in a
medium which shall be, as human milk is, alkaline.
This latter end is easily accomplished by the use
of a due amount of lime-water, and is justified by
the fact that it is a matter of experience, and almost
universally acknowledged as true, that it is a most
useful adjunct, rendering cows' milk more easy of
digestion by the human stomach.   The quantity
of lime-water to be used should be one-fourth of
the total by measure.   This may seem to many persons an excessive quantity, but when it is understood that if made as ordinarily directed, by agitating
water with lime and then filtering, it contains only
a very minute amount of lime, it becomes plain
that the use of lime-water means the administration
of a great deal of water and very little solid matter.

That the use of lime-water (alkali) in an infant
food makes a difference in its behavior with some
reagents is shown by the following experiments.
A food was made in the proportions which will
presently be given, and 10 c.c. of it agitated with
ether and alcohol, as directed in Chapter I, for the
extraction of the fat ; it was found that the coagulation took place in the form of a fine net-work,
which remained permanently distributed through

the lower stratum of the liquid, no sediment form-
ing at the bottom. When an exactly similar mixture was made, except that the lime-water was re-
placed with water, leaving the fluid acid, and this
agitated with ether and alcohol, thick, heavy curds
formed, which at once sank to the bottom. Again,
when two mixtures—one with and the other without lime-water—were treated with ten drops of
acetic acid, the one without lime-water showed
much larger, heavier coagula than that which contained lime-water. These experiments show with
certainty that the addition of lime-water does alter
the coagulability of the casein when experimented
with, whatever may take place in the stomach ; and
Lehmann's opinion has been already quoted, that the
acidity or alkalinity of milk makes a difference in
the formation of the coagulum. Whatever may be
the value of these artificial experiments, the great
reason for the use of lime-water is that the experience of man has found it good, and that is sufficient reason for its use in the present state of knowledge. It is quite possible that in the .future something better may be found, phosphate of lime, perhaps, for it is the salt which exists in milk in
larger quantity than any other ; but further and
exhaustive study of the inorganic constituents of
both human and cows' milk will be required to
place this matter upon an exact scientific basis. It
is very desirable that further study of the salts of
milk should be prosecuted, and it is much to be
hoped that in the near future exhaustive analyses

6

will be made. The amount of inorganic matter in cows' milk is so much greater than that in human milk that, as there is at present no means of removing it without altering or destroying the other component parts, no infant food can be made exactly like human milk in respect to the amount of salts contained.

So far as bringing the other proximate constituents to like proportions with those in human milk, the first step must be to so dilute with water as to get the desired quantity of casein ; the fat and sugar can be increased by the use of the necessary quantities of cream and commercial milk-sugar. Taking the averages of cream and good city milk as already given (see table), it will be found by calculation that if there be mixed together 10 c.c. of cream, 5 c.c. of milk, 10 c.c. of lime-water, and 15 c.c. of water, with 2.2 grams of milk-sugar, the desired mixture is had. That this is the case was not trusted to mere calculation, but an analysis of the mixture was made, both to verify the calculation and to observe how the mixture behaved when subjected to the analytic processes, whether it in its reactions more closely resembled cows' milk, with which it was made, or human milk. Table VIII shows the results obtained by such analyses.

The easiest way to prepare and use the food is as follows : There must be obtained from a reliable druggist packages of pure milk-sugar containing seventeen and three-quarters ($17\frac{3}{4}$) drachms each. The contents of one package is to be dissolved in a pint of water, and it is best to have a bottle which will contain just one pint, as there is then no need for further measuring. The contents of one of the sugar packages is put into the bottle, and when filled with water the sugar soon dissolves, and it is ready for use. The dry sugar keeps indefinitely, but after it is once dissolved it sours if kept more than a day or two in warm weather ; it is understood, therefore, that the sugar-water must be kept in a cool place, and if it should at any time become sour, which is easily discovered if it is smelled and tasted, it should be thrown out, and after the bottle has been carefully washed with boiling water, the contents of a fresh package dissolved. A milkman must be found who will serve good milk and cream, fresh every day. By good milk is meant ordinary milk, such as is easily procured in most cities, and not rich Jersey milk ; and in the same way the cream should be such as is ordinarily used in tea and coffee, and not the very rich cream of fancy cattle. The reason that ordinary milk and cream are recommended is because they are within the reach of almost every one, and not because they are any better than the rich milk of high-bred stock. If Jersey milk was to be used, it would be necessary to analyze specimens, and then make the necessary calculations as to how to dilute it to obtain the desired relative proportions of the proximate principles. When the child is to be fed, the nurse should mix together two (2) tablespoonfuls of cream, one (1) of milk, two (2) of lime-water, and three (3) of the sugar-water, and then, as soon as the mixture has been warmed, it may be poured into the bottle, and the food is ready for use. If the infant is healthy, this quantity will not satisfy it after the first few weeks, and then double the quantity must be prepared for each feeding. Twice as many table-spoonfuls of each of the ingredients must be mixed together, making sixteen tablespoonfuls (about half a pint) in all.

This food should not be given any stronger until the child is eight or nine months old, at least; but if the infant is a healthy one, it may take as much of it as it wants, but always of the same strength. A robust infant will often take three pints, or even more, in each twenty-four hours. It is an easy matter for any one to learn how to make lime-water; and it is advisable to have it made at home, for a great deal is used, and if it is made at home much trouble and expense are saved.

Table VIII shows the proportions in which the various proximate constituents exist in different kinds of milk, and of cream, and of foods.

With regard to the amount of food taken by a . healthy infant there has been much disagreement, and the same is the case with the question of the propriety of increasing, from week to week, the strength of any artificial food given to infants. Most authorities have advised that the artificial foods should be increased in concentration until finally, if cows' milk was used, it should be given pure. The propriety of this procedure during the earlier

TABLE VIII.

	Human. (Mean composition from milk of 43 women.)	Artificial Food: Cream, 10 c.c.; milk 5 c.c.; lime-water, 10 c.c.; water, 15 c.c.; sugar, 2.2 grams. (Cream contained 12.470 per cent. of Fat.)	Artificial Food: Cream, 2 table-spoonfuls; milk, 1 do.; lime-water, 2 do.; sugar-water, 3 do. (Cream contained 17.129 per cent. Fat. Each tablespoonful was 20 c.c. Sugar-water was 17¾ drachms to pint.)	Cows' Milk.	Cows' Milk.	Eagle Brand Condensed Milk.	Condensed, 1 teaspoonful (10.233 grams) to 6 table-spoonfuls (90 c.c.) of Water.	Cream.	Cream.	Creams.	Amount of Fat in Each.
Water......	87.163	88.357	87.639	88.549	87.012	27.942	92.673	79.122	79.901	No. 1	19.020
Fat........	4.283	3.506	4.765	3.310	4.209	10.335	1.095	13.362	12.470	" 2	17.507
Casein....	1.046	1.214	1.115	2.792	3.252	9.522	.868	2.919	2.846	" 3	13.362
Sugar......	7.407	6.669	6.264	4.898	5.000	50.861	5.206	4.140	4.308	" 4	12.470
Ash........	.101	.254	.217	.451	.527	1.340	.158	.457	.475	" 5	17.129
										" 6	16.024
										" 7	13.825
										" 8	14.950
										" 9	18.082
										" 10	16.502
										" 11	12.159
										" 12	15.611
										" 13	19.071
										" 14	11.782
										" 15	18.519
										" 16	21.465
										" 17	21.290
Total......	100.000	100.000	100.000	100.000	100.000	100.000	100.000	100.000	100.000	Average from the 17, 16.398.	
Error.......	.009 per cent. loss.	.009 per cent. loss.	.029 per cent. in excess.	.029 per cent. in excess.	.058 per cent. loss.	.476 per cent. loss.	.009 per cent. in excess.	.109 per cent. loss.	.039 per cent. in excess.		

The human milk average is the result of ten analyses made. Eight separate analyses were made of the milk of different women; on another occasion, equal quantities of milk were taken from twenty-seven (27) women, and a portion of this analyzed; on a third, equal quantities of milk were taken from eight (8) colored women, and this subjected to analysis.

months of life is very doubtful. Although there is some authority for believing that the amount of the solid ingredients in human milk increases from month to month as lactation goes on, such an opinion should be accepted only with great caution, for it seems likely that if there is any increase in the concentration of the milk after the colostrum has once disappeared, and the nursing process has settled into its even course, the increase is so slight that it may be disregarded. Analyses show that the milk of a woman whose child is two months old does not differ materially from that of one whose child is twelve or fifteen months old. If, then, nature has made no difference, which our means of analysis will detect, between the milk of a woman who has been nursing two months and one who has nursed twelve, an artificial food which has been found to suit an infant at two months should be made more concentrated only very gradually, and with careful observation of the effect upon the health of the infant. It is best, therefore, if the infant thrives and grows as it should, *not* to make any change in the food until after six to nine months of age have been attained.

The amount of milk secreted in twenty four hours by a healthy woman has been variously estimated at from one to ninety-two fluidounces. Lehmann* quotes Lampérierre, who used an apparatus of his own invention, having artificial lips, gums, and teeth,

---

* *Loc. cit.*

to draw the milk from the breast, as authority for believing that as much as forty-one ounces (1,320 grams) are often secreted in twenty-four hours. He found, after drawing the milk of a large number of women, that about fifty to sixty grams were secreted by each breast in the course of two hours.

Parrot* followed a method proposed by Natalis Guillot, which was to weigh an infant immediately before and after each nursing, and the increment in weight gave the amount of milk taken. Guillot weighed an infant only once ·a day, and assuming that it nursed about twenty-five times a day, concluded that the amount of milk taken was, on the second day after birth, twenty-two ounces (675 grams), and on the eighteenth day, ninety-two ounces (2,975 grams). Parrot considers this estimate as much too high, and quotes Bouchaud, who estimated the quantity by weighing directly before and after each nursing. By this method it was determined that an infant nursed only from eight to ten times daily, and the following results were arrived at as to the quantities of milk taken from the first day after birth up to nine months :—

First day	30 grams (7½ drachms).
Second day	150 " (4½ oz.).
Third day	450 " (14 ").
Fourth day	550 " (17 ").
From the first to the third month	640 " (20 ").
From the third to the fourth month	750 " (23½ ").
From the fourth to the sixth month	850 " (27½ ").
From the sixth to the ninth month	950 " (30½ ").

* *Clinique des Nouveau-Nés, L'Athrepsie,* page 431.

Parrot says of these figures that he accepts them as correct after having made experiments himself to test their precision. Speaking of the article of Biedert, Parrot says he cannot agree with him, and thinks that in the great majority of cases it is best to give infants pure cows' milk even from the beginning, and that in exceptional cases, if the milk has to be diluted, only one-third part of water should be added. Pure cows' milk, he says, should be given, and in quantities as follows :—

First day	5	drachms (20 grams).
Second day	3	ounces (100 ").
Third day	9½	" (300 ").
Fourth day	13½	" (434 ").
From the first to the third month	14½	" (460 ").
From the third to the fourth month	14½	" (460 ").
From the fourth to the sixth month	17½	" (566 ").
From the sixth to the ninth month	20	" (634 ").

Not being certain that the above quoted figures were exactly correct, Parrot determined to test their accuracy by estimating by Bouchaud's process the amount of food taken by healthy hand-fed infants, weighing them before and after each feeding. Twelve healthy infants of various ages were selected, and were fed with pure cows' milk, which was given them six times daily, with the following results :—

First day,	1 infant	5¼ ounces (167 grams).
Second day,	3 infants (mean)	4½ " (148 ").
Third day,	3 " "	5½ " (179 ").
Fourth day,	2 " "	7½ " (238 ").

Fifth day,	2 infants (mean)	....	7	ounces	(222 grams).
Eleventh day, 2	"	"	 5	"	(158 ").
First month, 2	"	"	 8	"	(257 ").
Second month, 2	"	"	.... 12½	"	(400 ").
Sixth month, 2	"	"	 22	"	(708 ").

If the last two tables are compared, he says, it will be seen that the results are, in all essentials, thè same, although there are minor differences.

It is difficult to estimate the value of the results attained by this method; but they are not so conclusive as those given by Dr. J. Forsyth Meigs,* who speaks of the matter as follows : " I have found very few statements by medical writers as to the quantity of milk furnished by nursing-women, and the few that I have found differ so much from each other that I deem them of very moderate value. . . .

" My own observations amount to only three in number; but the mode of determination of the amount of milk yielded in each case was so necessarily exact, that I have entire faith in their accuracy so far as they go. The milk was drawn from the breasts by a breast-pump in each case, and then accurately measured.

" The first observation was made some thirty years since. A healthy woman, whose mother was a monthly nurse, was confined of a still-born child.

---

* *The Sanitary Care and Treatment of Children and their Diseases,* by Drs. Elizabeth Garrett-Anderson, Samuel C. Busey, A. Jacobi, J. Forsyth Meigs, and J. Lewis Smith, prepared by request of the Trustees of the Thomas Wilson Sanitarium of Baltimore. Boston, 1881.

The flow of milk was kept up by means of a young puppy. At the end of six weeks she obtained a place as wet-nurse, and the day before she went to her place, I had all the milk her breasts furnished for twenty-four hours drawn with a good breast-pump. It measured exactly a quart. I measured it myself. Is it not reasonable to suppose that, had the breast-glands been stimulated in this woman in the natural method, to wit, by the maternal instinct and by the suction of a healthy child, the amount would have been larger—say three pints? Since that period, I have had two admirable opportunities for determining exactly the amount of milk supplied by a healthy woman. In one case, a child four months old, suddenly, owing to a long illness from a chronic suppuration, weaned itself from its mother. It was fed for a time on cows' milk, with Mellin's food ; but becoming very ill, I sent for a wet-nurse. The child could not be induced to take the breast, and the milk was, therefore, drawn by a breast-pump, and fed to the child from an ordinary nursing-bottle. The wet-nurse's child was at this time two months old. At first only small quantities, one or two ounces, were retained ; but after several days the child took daily of this milk as much as thirty-six ounces. Besides this quantity, which was drawn regularly by the breast-pump, the nurse suckled her own child in part. Assuming that she gave her own child a pint, we find that the amount supplied by her was fully three pints, or forty-eight ounces daily.

"In the second case, a child born of a very

healthy young woman, was unable to nurse because of a congenital defect of the mouth. The milk was drawn by a breast-pump, and administered from a sucking-bottle. When the child was five and six weeks old, it was taking eighteen and twenty-three ounces per day. But, at the same time, the quantity drawn each day from the breasts, accurately measured, was $39\frac{3}{4}$, 41, $33\frac{1}{4}$, 39, $39\frac{1}{4}$, $39\frac{1}{4}$, $31\frac{1}{4}$, $41\frac{1}{2}$, $44\frac{1}{2}$, 35, 40, and $39\frac{1}{4}$ ounces. The largest amount any one day, in this case, was, therefore, $44\frac{1}{2}$, and the smallest $31\frac{1}{4}$ ounces. Is it not probable that, had the breasts been stimulated in the natural way in this woman, the quantity would have been greater rather than less ? "

These observations prove conclusively that the amount of milk supplied in a day by a woman is in excess of what is commonly supposed. In no one of the three instances mentioned was the child more than two months old; and although in the two instances in which the milk was given to an infant, in neither was the whole quantity taken, yet it must be remembered that one infant was very ill and the other had a cleft palate. It would seem fair, then, to conclude that if the infants had been healthy, their demands would have been equal to the supply, and three pints of milk taken instead of about two.

With regard to the use of condensed milk as a food for young infants, it cannot be recommended. It is sometimes very useful when fresh milk is not available ; and occasionally, when children are sick, they will take and digest it when they cannot take other things, and under such circumstances it should be used, but such cases are very exceptional. The only explanation of the great success it has met with, and the large extent to which it is used, is in the fact that when it is mixed, as is usually done in this city, in the proportion of one teaspoonful to six tablespoonfuls of water, it contains (see Table VIII) much more nearly the same percentage of casein that is found in human milk than does any other commonly used food. That is to say, it is cows' milk much more diluted than the usually employed fresh-milk mixtures, and with a much larger quantity of sugar. This explains why it is so often well digested; for, as has been already said, it is the excessive quantity of casein in cows' milk that infants are unable to digest. At the same time, a consideration of the composition of this condensed-milk mixture, and an understanding that it contains a very much less proportion of fat and less sugar than does human milk, affords an adequate explanation of the fact that children who are fed for many months exclusively upon condensed milk so often fail to thrive.

The weight of testimony that condensed milk is by no means so perfect a food for infants as has been supposed by many physicians is year by year accumulating. Dr. W. D. Booker* says of the children remaining at the Thomas Wilson Sanitarium for long periods during the summer of 1884,

* *Fifth Annual Report of the Thomas Wilson Sanitarium for Children of Baltimore City.* 1885. Page 12.

" out of thirty-seven suffering with entero-colitis, under one year of age, only six nursed exclusively at the breast. Only one of the six was seriously sick with bowel trouble at any time. Eleven children had the breast-milk and artificial food together, whilst twenty had artificial food alone. Those who nursed in part from the breast suffered almost as much as those fed exclusively upon artificial food. Of the twenty fed on artificial food, sixteen were seriously sick. Six of the eleven raised on breast-milk and artificial food together were seriously sick.

" The artificial food given previously to their coming to the Sanitarium varied from condensed milk, cows' milk, and oatmeal water, to anything on the parents' table. *A larger number* of those seriously sick had been fed upon condensed milk than any other article."

In the article on Food (*Diseases of Children*, Meigs & Pepper, Phila., 1882), the question of the advantages and disadvantages of condensed milk is pretty fully discussed, and quite a number of cases given and authorities quoted, and an opinion expressed adverse to its general use as a food for young infants.

There appear only two possible reasons why condensed milk should be better than fresh milk as a food for infants—one that it has been cooked, and the other, that there has been a large amount of cane-sugar added. When it is considered that these possible advantages are offset by the facts that fresh milk may easily be cooked (if there is any virtue in

the process), and sugar added to any extent that
may be desired, and that the honesty of the manu-
facturer must be entirely depended upon for the
purity of the article offered for sale, and that it may
have been kept for a very long time ; a time must
come when condensed milk will cease to hold the
place it now does in this community as an article of
food for young infants.   It must be that it holds its
present high reputation because, as has been already
stated, it is given dilute, and the quantity of casein
is therefore small; and that with a better understanding of the relative compositions of human and
cows' milk among physicians, and a better use of
fresh cows' milk, condensed milk must find its
proper level, and cease to be used except when fresh
milk is unavailable, or as a temporary substitute in
cases of disease when other foods are found not to be
well digested.

CHAPTER VI.

CONCLUSION.

To sum up the advice which has been given throughout this book, but which is scattered here and there with the reasons upon which are based the various conclusions, it may be said that the author deems it best, if a child is to be hand-fed from birth, that it should be given the food which is described at page 74, and that this should not be increased in strength until after the child is at least from six to nine months of age. If, however, the case to be dealt with is that of an older infant that has been fed upon other things, and is sick or ill-nourished, it will probably not be so easily managed; for the child will have acquired some power of taste, and will refuse to take what is not agreeable to it, and will, besides, almost certainly have some impairment of its digestive functions. If the case be one of an infant under six or nine months of age, the mixture should be tried, and often does well if it is taken. One of the difficulties to be overcome in most cases is that the foods previously used have been very sweet, and to get the child to take any food a large amount of sugar must be added. This can generally be overcome by giving the large amount of sugar to suit the taste for a time, and then gradually, in the course of a week or two, cutting it down

until the desired amount only is taken. Another
difficulty in making any change of food is that all
persons are naturally impatient, and will not wait long
enough to really ascertain whether what is being
tried is suitable or not, but are disposed to change
from one thing to another every few days, before
any one of them has been given a fair trial. When
an infant has been sick and has its digestion dis-
ordered, it cannot show much improvement in less
than several days or a week, no matter what food is
given.

In artificially feeding a child of nine months to
a year old, the mixture recommended by Dr. J.
Forsyth Meigs, of two tablespoonfuls of milk,
cream, lime-water, and arrowroot-water (a teaspoonful of arrowroot to a pint of boiling water) each,
and a little sugar, will often be found to suit well,
or the mixture of milk and barley-water recommended by Dr. Jacobi (*Hygiene, etc.*, by Buck, *loc.
cit.*). A sick child of this age should be fed about
every two hours, and only a small quantity at a
time should be given ; and the physician who shows
the greatest fertility of resource in finding what the
particular child can take and assimilate is the best
for the case, for, as Dr. J. Forsyth Meigs (*Sanitary
Care and Treatment of Children, loc. cit.*, page 231)
well says, " children, like adults, are a law to themselves, and he is the successful physician who dis-
covers the law of each patient, and so is enabled to
carry him through some special crisis of his life."

It is a good plan, and one which should in all

cases be followed out, whether a child is nursed or hand-fed, that it should be taught to drink from a small cup when it is two or three months old; this is easily managed with a little persistence, for, although the child will splutter and spill more over its bib than it drinks when the attempt is first made, yet after from one to three weeks' trial it will be found that children almost always learn to drink, and like it, and it need not at all interfere with their using a bottle or nursing from the breast the rest of the day. At first only water should be given, and that once a day; but after the child has learned to drink, and is three months old, if it is nursed it is a good thing to give it once a day three or four ounces of artificial food. This plan is good, both because it gives the mother a respite from the very confining duties of nursing, and because it is well for the child to learn to digest something else beside breast-milk. Besides which, if anything happens to the mother, the infant is able, if the necessity arise, to take other nourishment than breast-milk; it will also be found a much easier matter to wean the infant when the time comes, if it has already been accustomed to take artificial food; lastly, the process of weaning is much less likely to produce any disturbance of health.

After infants are from one year to eighteen months of age, they are generally able to digest pure cows' milk, and the attempt should be made to give it to them, the strength of whatever artificial food they have been taking being gradually increased until at

7

last the pure milk is given. This should be done, of course, with due caution, and if it is found that the digestion of the child will not bear the increase, the old mixture, whatever it may have been, which has previously suited, should be given again, and the attempt to strengthen the food not made for a few weeks or a month or two, as the case may be.

Children under two years of age are generally best fed upon milk and milk foods, and the less this is departed from, as a rule, the better. Under this age they should never be taken to the table, for it only gives the child the fancy for articles of diet which, if it never saw, it would not want. It is well to give young infants nothing but their regular food, and not to give pieces of cake or candy, or anything else of the kind, for the pleasure of seeing them enjoy it. If this rule is observed, parents save themselves a great deal of annoyance in their children's crying for what they cannot have.

In the great majority of cases children have not much desire for animal food of any sort until after the first dentition is over, unless the craving is fostered in them by their being given one thing and another to eat, and thus there is created what is almost an unnatural appetite. If a child is well and thrives, taking plenty of milk, no great effort should be made to induce it to take other articles of diet until after the processes of the first dentition are completed. This is, of course, not intended to be an absolute rule, for many children want and seem to need, after the first year, a meal once or twice a

day of something beside milk and bread. After
the first year there may often with advantage be
given for the mid-day meal some soup, or boiled
rice, or potato with butter and salt or a little meat-
gravy upon it. For breakfast, a soft-boiled or
poached egg, oatmeal with milk and sugar, wheaten
grits, or hominy. A little finely-cut meat for din-
ner suits many children. They may take at all
times, after the first year, as much bread and butter and crackers as they want; but, as a general
rule, the diet should be very simple, and fruits,
cakes, and made dishes of all sorts should be avoided.

No mother should feel uneasy if her child takes
almost nothing but milk and bread and butter until
after it is two years of age, if only it takes plenty of
them, and continues well and develops naturally;
nor should any great effort be made to induce it to
take meat and other things when it evinces no
appetite for them or repugnance to them, under
the idea that it is not getting sufficient nourishment.
Children will often live thus until they are two
years old or a little more, and then gradually begin to want and eat other things. No child ever
yet grew up eating only milk and bread, so if
parents and physicians will have patience and wait,
the child will surely begin to eat like other people.

The times at which children should be fed, and
the amounts to be given, are not easy to fix; for
each child is so different from every other one that
what suits one is bad for another, each one being
more or less of a rule by itself. Still, however,

general advice can be given, which must be modi-
fied to meet the demands of each particular case.

Infants have their idiosyncrasies which show
themselves at once, although this may seem hard
to believe. The author knows two children, one of
whom, from the hour of his birth, always was a
slow eater; in nursing he would draw once or twice
at the breast, and then let go and roll his head
about for awhile, then with persuasion would again
take hold, and after taking another mouthful or two,
the same process would be repeated. He would
seldom take less than three-quarters of an hour at
each nursing. A second child, born a little less
than fourteen months afterward of the same parents,
would always nurse vigorously and continuously
until he had all he required, and then nothing
would induce him to take another drop; and it seldom took more than a quarter of an hour for him
to nurse. These children are now five and six years
old, and they eat exactly as they nursed from the
very day of their birth ; the one plays with his food,
looks about, talks, and takes the longest time to
eat his meals ; the other begins, eats rapidly and
vigorously for a short time, and then will push back
his plate, and no persuasion will induce him to eat
more. These instances show how infants are born
with their individualities, and therefore it must be
remembered that all rules must be bent to suit each
particular case ; and for this reason the quantity of
food that is proper for one child will not be exactly
what another needs ; and if one child needs to be fed

five times a day, perhaps another will require food six or seven times.

Infants do not seem to need much food, nor need it be very often given, during the first three days after birth; after that time, however, they should have nourishment about every two or three hours; and this will be the case with the night as well as the day during the first few weeks of life. After three or four weeks they will not require nourishment so often during the night. Between ten and six, if they are nursed or fed twice, say about at one and again at four, it is usually sufficient, and some infants will even nurse only once. When an infant is six weeks to two months old, it will usually require nourishment about every three hours during the day and once or twice during the night, that is, between ten at night and six in the morning. During the second, third, and even the fourth months of life infants are not usually troublesome; they eat at regular times and sleep well and soundly, but after this period, usually during the fourth month of life, the processes of dentition begin, and many infants become very irregular in their habits, sleeping at all sorts of times and often very little. No one knows so well as a mother who has had children what actual tortures they often have to endure during this period; infants will be awake almost the whole night for weeks at a time. They seem to live without sleep for long periods, like the insane, and as soon as night comes on they are preternaturally wide awake.

A child of from nine to twelve months old will require to be fed at about six to seven in the morning, at eleven, at three, at six to seven, at half-past ten, and once in the night; or often five times in the twenty-four hours will be found sufficient. Most children will demand to be fed once during the night until they are between eighteen months and two and a half years of age, according to the individuality of the child, and somewhat according to the disposition of the mother to indulge it; for, as with all other habits, it is usually a little troublesome to break up the custom of a midnight meal, although, if it is properly gone about, there is generally no great difficulty; and it is a good thing to teach a child to sleep through the night without food.

During the first month of life, an infant will take at each feeding or nursing about one to four ounces of nourishment; and they should be given each time enough to satisfy them. If a child is hand-fed, the bottle used should hold eight ounces ; and although during the first two or three months only four to six ounces at each feeding will usually be taken, after the age of six or eight months has been reached they will usually take the whole eight ounces, and sometimes a little more. Between three months of age and one year, children will generally take from two pints or a little less, to three a day.

The food which has been recommended in this work, and which is carefully described in a previous chapter, was the result of a study of the subject both from a theoretical and practical stand-point. It had been found by experience and experiment that about such a mixture of milk and cream as was recommended by Dr. J. Forsyth Meigs (see page 88) was digested by the infant stomach better than any other food, except human breast-milk ; and then a careful study of the relative composition of human and cows' milk led to the concoction of the food in which the various constituents are mixed as nearly as possible in the same proportions as they exist in human milk. This food has been quite extensively tested by the author, and in all instances in which it has been tried thus far, it has proved successful. It has been used where condensed milk had failed, for infants that were partially nursed and partially hand-fed, for entirely artificially-fed children, in cases of disease and of malnutrition, and, as already said, it has seemed to be wonderfully useful and easily digested. Of course, no food has been found, or ever will be found, so good as the nourishment which a healthy mother is able to give her child, and the food recommended will sometimes fail, as all things fail ; still, in the opinion of the author, it is much more nearly what is wanted than anything previously recommended, being founded upon both theory and practical observation and experiment.

BIBLIOGRAPHY.

Foods; Composition and Analysis. A. W. Blyth. London, 1882.
Practical Hygiene, by E. A. Parkes. London, 1873.
Milk Analysis. J. Alfred Wanklyn. New York, 1874.
Analysis of Milk, Condensed Milk, and Infants' Milk-Foods, by Dr. N. Gerber. New York, 1882.
The Practitioner, May, 1882. On the insufficient use of milk as an article of food in England, by Dyce Duckworth.
Chemistry for Medical Students, by William Odling.
German Clinical Lectures. 2d Series. New Sydenham Society Translation. The Food of Infants, by Prof. F. A. Kehrer.
Sanitary Care and Treatment of Children. Being a Series of Five Essays, by Drs. Elizabeth Garret-Anderson, Samuel C. Busey, A. Jacobi, J. Forsyth Meigs, and J. Lewis Smith.
Clinique des Nouveau-Nés, L'Athrepsie, par J. Parrot. Paris, 1877.
Lehrbuch der Physiologischen Chemie, von Dr. E. F. v. Gorup-Besanez. Braunschweig, 1867.
Virchow's Archiv für patholog. Anat., etc. Bd. lx, 1874. Neue Untersuchungen und klinische Beobachtungen über Menschen- und Kuhmilch als Kindernahrungsmittel, von Dr. Ph. Biedert.
Journal de Pharmacie, Tome 25. Mémoire sur le lait, par MM. O. Henri et A. Chevallier.
Journal de Pharmacie, Tome 25. Concernant l'analyse du lait, par M. Le Canu.
Annales d'Hygiéne Publique et de Médicine Légale, Tome 26, 1841. Mémoire sur le Lait, par T. A. Quevenne.
The Lancet, 1871. Vol. I. On a Rapid and Accurate Method of Milk Analysis, by John Muter.
The Lancet, 1871. Vol. I. On Human Milk, by C. Meynott Tidy.
London Hospital Reports, 1867. On Human Milk, by C. Meynott Tidy.
Document 38—1885. City of Boston. Twenty-sixth Annual Report of the Milk Inspector. Bennett F. Davenport, M.D.
Fifth Annual Report of the Thomas Wilson Sanitarium for Children of Baltimore. Baltimore, 1885.
Histoire des Enfants Abandonnés, par Ernest Semichon. Paris, 1880.
La Vérité sur les Enfants Trouvés, par le Dr. Brochard. Paris, 1876.

Histoire Administrative de l'œuvre des Enfants Trouvés abandonnés et orphelins de Lyon, par E. Fayard. Paris, 1873.

L'Enfance a Paris, par Le Vicomte D'Haussonville. Paris, 1879.

Foods, by Edward Smith. New York, 1873.

Journal of the Franklin Institute, April, 1882. Milk, by Reuben Haines.

Diseases of Children, by Meigs and Pepper. Philadelphia, 1882.

Traité de Chimie Pathologique, par Becquerel et Rodier. Paris, 1854.

Untersuchungen über die Chemischen Unterschiede der Menschen- und Kuhmilch, von Dr. Ph. Biedert. Stuttgart, 1884.

Virchow's Archiv für pathologische, etc. Bd. xci, 1883. Milch-Analyse und das Menschen- und Kuhcasein, von Dr. Ph. Biedert.

Deutschen Medicinischen Wochenschrift, No. 3, 1883. Ueber rein diätetische Behandlung der Ernährungskrankheiten der Säuglinge, von Dr. Ph. Biedert.

Archives of Medicine, October, 1882. A Contribution to the Study of Anæmia, by F. P. Henry.

The Medical News, November 4, 1882. The Artificial Feeding of Infants, by Arthur V. Meigs.

Philadelphia Medical Times, July 1, 1882. Milk Analysis, by Arthur V. Meigs.

Proceedings of the Philadelphia County Medical Society, Vol. VI, 1883-4, page 92. Proof that Human Milk contains only about One Per Cent. of Casein ; with Remarks upon Infant Feeding, by Arthur V. Meigs.

Transactions of the College of Physicians of Philadelphia. Third series, Vol. VI, page 377. Infant Foods, by Professor Albert R. Leeds, PH.D.

Transactions of the College of Physicians of Philadelphia. Third Series, Vol. VII, page 225. The Composition and Methods of Analysis of Human Milk, by Professor Albert R. Leeds, PH.D.

Transactions of the College of Physicians of Philadelphia. Third Series, Vol. VIII, page 139. A Criticism of Dr. Leeds' Paper on " The Composition and Methods of Analysis of Human Milk."

Littell's Living Age, No. 2140, June 27, 1885. From the Nineteenth Century, Diet in Relation to Age and Activity, by Sir Henry Thompson.

The American Medical Weekly, New York, January 7, 1882. Highly Important and Extensively Advertised Cereal Foods under the Microscope, etc., by Ephraim Cutter, A.M., M.D.

Public Ledger, of Philadelphia, January 1, 1884. Census Report.

Medical News, November 25, 1882. Mortality Statistics of the United States.

American Journal of Pharmacy, October 1, 1874. The Chemistry of Milk, by Ed. J. Hallock.

Water Analysis, by J. Alfred Wanklyn and Ernest Theophron Chapman. London, 1876.

INDEX.